Mechanisms and Management of Cardiac

A~~rrhythmias~~

Clif

Professe
Manch
Manch

First published in 2001
by BMJ Books, BMA House, Tavistock Square,
London WC1H 9JR

www.bmjbooks.com

British Library Cataloguing in Publication Data
A catalogue record for this book is available from the British Library

ISBN 0-7279-1194-5

Typeset by Newgen Imaging Systems (P) Ltd., Chennai, India
Printed and Bound by Selwood Printing Ltd, Burgess Hill, West Sussex

To Lucy

Contents

Preface

My interest in cardiac arrhythmias stems from my time as a clinical medical student and house physician at St Bartholomew's Hospital in London. A combination of the logical basis to therapy (at least relative to most other medical disciplines) and the dramatic successes of some forms of treatment drew me to the subject. I remember being surprised to find that, although clinical textbooks on arrhythmia management would usually have a section on "basic electrophysiology" or "the action potential", there was invariably no attempt made to explain the clinical arrhythmias in these terms. Similarly, accounts of the ionic processes underlying activation of cardiac cells would include a discussion of clinical arrhythmias as an afterthought if at all. There have been dramatic advances in both fields since that time. My impression is that this divide remains despite the recent publication of several large multiauthored texts which address both areas in a single volume. The aim of this monograph is to provide medical students, house physicians, and cardiologists in training with a logical, scientifically based framework for the management of arrhythmias in which the relevant aspects of basic electrophysiology are put in the clinical context. The fundamental concepts introduced in the first three chapters are expanded and illustrated in subsequent sections. Thereafter each arrhythmia is discussed in greater detail with particular emphasis on mechanism, clinical setting, and long term or definitive therapy. Finally the principles of clinical management of arrhythmias are addressed, with chapters on presentation, acute diagnosis and therapy, antiarrhythmic drugs, ablation techniques, and implantable cardioverter defibrillators.

I would like to acknowledge my clinician teachers and colleagues, especially John Camm, Adam Fitzpatrick, Michael Griffith, Edward Rowland, and David Ward for their ideas and advice which are contained in this volume. Finally, I am grateful to Maurits Allessie for an inspiring apprenticeship in experimental electrophysiology and to the British Heart Foundation for allowing me to spend a year in his laboratory in Maastricht.

PART I
CELLULAR AND TISSUE ELECTROPHYSIOLOGY

1: Ion channels and ion currents

Each of the cells of the human body is surrounded by a lipid membrane and, whilst many particles can slowly cross these membranes by diffusion, most life processes in higher organisms could not occur without more effective and regulated mechanisms for the transfer of molecules into and out of cells. Ion channels are integral membrane proteins that are responsible for rapid transmembrane flow of millions of charged particles per second thereby generating electrical impulses in the excitable tissues of brain, nerve, heart, and muscle. The importance of these structures is highlighted by the fact that some cells use up to 50% of their energy expenditure maintaining gradients of ions across their membranes. Despite evidence of a great diversity of different channels within individuals and between species, the basic structure of these proteins is remarkably well conserved and voltage-sensitive sodium, calcium, and potassium channels appear to be members of a closely related gene family (Figure 1.1).

General properties of ion channels

Ion channels show ion selectivity, in that they usually allow only one type of ion to pass. They can be either open or closed (gating), depending upon either the electric field across the membrane (voltage-gated), the time relative to a previous channel event (time-dependent), or the presence of an appropriate molecule (ligand-gated). The voltage-gated and time-dependent currents associated with these channels are discussed in more detail below. Examples of ligand-gated channels are the potassium channels which open or close in response to acetylcholine and ATP ($I_{K(ACh)}$ and $I_{K(ATP)}$ respectively). Ion channel gating mechanisms are usually discussed in relation to a mathematical model of the action potential devised by Hodgkin and Huxley in 1952–3. In this model, passage of sodium ions is determined by three "m" gates on the extracellular side of the channel and one "h" gate on the intracellular side (Figure 1.2). Between each action potential the m gates are closed and the h gates open (resting state). Depolarisation (see below) causes the m gates to open and the h gate to close (voltage dependence) but the closure of the h gate is slightly later than the m gate opening. Consequently both gates are open for a short period of time, sodium ions rush into the cell, and the action potential is initiated.

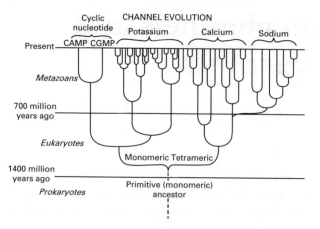

Figure 1.1 Evolution of the family of channel proteins. Near the end of the Archeozoic period, when eukaryotes evolved from the prokaryotes, a primitive monomeric channel protein is believed to have given rise to the non-covalently linked subunits of potassium and cyclic nucleotide-gated channels, and to tetrameric calcium channels. Later, during the Cambrian period, tetrameric sodium channels are thought to have evolved from the calcium channels. There appear to be many more potassium channel subtypes than subtypes of the calcium channel: evidence that there are even fewer sodium channel subtypes is consistent with their more recent evolution. (*From* Katz AM. Ion channels and cardiology: the need for bridges across a widening boundary. In: Spooner PM, Brown AM, eds. *Ion channels in the cardiovascular system*. Aronk, NY: Futura Publishing, 1994.)

Following inactivation, the gates return to their resting state. This model has been refined in recent years but the basic concepts appear to hold true. Although the opening of single channels as described above is an "all or nothing" phenomenon, the total current flowing into the cell is dependent upon the current through an individual channel, the number of channels in the cell, and the probability of each channel being open.

Molecular structure of cardiac ion channels

The basic structure of an ion channel is one of a group of protein subunits embedded within the cell membrane in such a way as to form a central hydrophilic pore through which ions can pass.

Sodium channels

The sodium channel consists of alpha (central component) and beta (subsidiary) subunits. Each alpha subunit has four homologous domains, linked by covalent bonds, which wrap around the central pore region, and each domain can be considered as contributing 25% of the wall of the channel pore (Figure 1.3A). The domains are made up of six helical protein segments (S1–S6), all of which traverse the cell membrane (Figure 1.3B). Attempts have been made to determine the likely function of each segment in terms of

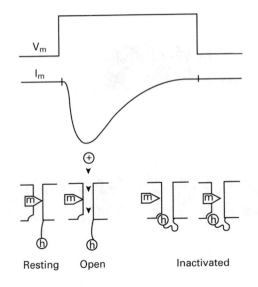

Figure 1.2   Proposed role of the m and h gating mechanisms in current flow through the Na$^+$ channel. *Top and middle*: representations of a step change in membrane potential Vm and the resulting current Im. *Lower*: ion channel movement through the channel is controlled by activation (m) and inactivation (h) gates (see text). (*From* Grant AO. Sodium channel blockade as an antiarrhythmic mechanism. In: Breithardt G, Borggrefe M, Camm J, Shenasa M, eds. *Antiarrhythmic drugs*. Berlin: Springer, 1994.)

the known physiological properties of the sodium channel. The region between S5 and S6 of each segment is thought to form the pore itself. The S4 segment, unlike the other segments, is positively charged and is considered a good candidate for the voltage sensor or m gate. The short segment linking S6 of domain III and S1 of domain IV is identified as a possible candidate for the h gate that is involved in channel inactivation, possibly by means of a "hinged lid" mechanism of occluding the pore (see Figure 1.2). The presence of the beta subunit has a modulating effect on the alpha subunit such that activation and inactivation of sodium channels are accelerated by its presence. Abnormalities of the sodium channel underlie some forms of the long QT syndrome and also the Brugada syndrome (see Chapters 11 and 12).

Potassium channels

Some voltage-gated potassium channels (termed "shaker-related" because of their abnormal expression in a fruit fly mutant that shakes its legs when exposed to ether) show striking structural similarity to the sodium channel in that the pore is formed from an association of four protein structures. These structures are not covalently bonded, however, but form a non-covalent association: hence they are referred to as alpha subunits rather than domains (Figure 1.4). These subunits are structurally very similar to the sodium channel domains, each consisting of six segments: the S4 segment and P

5

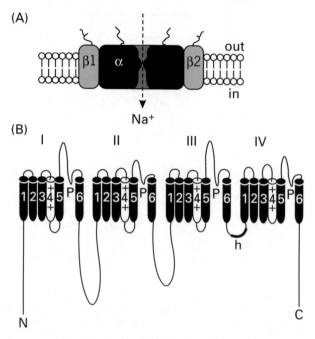

Figure 1.3   Structure of the voltage-gated Na$^+$ channel. (*From* Jalife J, Delmar M, Davidenko JM, Anumonwo JMB. *Basic cardiac electrophysiology for the clinician.* Armonk, NY: Futura, 1999.)

region (S5–S6) are present and probably play similar roles of voltage sensing and ion permeation as in the sodium channel. Potassium channels are thought to undergo inactivation by means of the physical plugging of the intracellular mouth of the channel with a particle formed by the N-terminal by what is termed the "ball and chain" mechanism. As well as this N-type inactivation, some potassium channels show C-type inactivation which involves the occlusion of the external mouth of the channel pore. The delayed rectifier currents I_{Kr} and I_{Ks} occur through shaker-type channels, as does the transient inward current (I_{TI}). I_{Kr} is encoded by the human ether-a-go-go related gene (HERG) localised on chromosome 7 and the channel protein underlying I_{Ks} is thought to be formed by the coassembly of a shaker-type channel protein and the minK protein. Mutations in the genes encoding these proteins are responsible for various forms of the congenital long QT syndrome (see Chapter 12). Unlike the shaker potassium channels, the inward rectifier potassium channels (I_{K1}) have only two transmembrane segments (M1 and M2), similar to the shaker S5 and S6 segments and pore region: the pore is thought to be formed by a tetrameric assembly.

Calcium channels

The calcium channel consists of multiple subunits: two alpha, one each of beta, gamma, delta. The alpha subunit forms the pore and the role of the

(A)

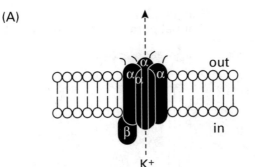

(B)

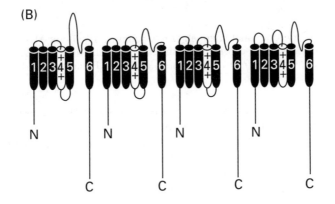

Figure 1.4   Structure of the shaker-related K^+ channel. (*From* Jalife J, Delmar M, Davidenko JM, Anumonwo JMB. *Basic cardiac electrophysiology for the clinician.* Armonk, NY: Futura, 1999.)

other subunits remains unclear. Remarkable homology exists between the alpha 1 subunit of the L-type calcium channel and the pore-forming alpha subunit of voltage-dependent sodium channels, both having four homologous domains composed of six transmembrane segments each. The S4 segment again is likely to be involved in activation gating. The loop between domains 2 and 3 is thought to be important in excitation contraction coupling.

As well as being controlled in the short term by voltage- and time-dependent mechanisms, ion channel conductance is modulated over longer time periods by protein phosphorylation and molecular interaction with guanine nucleotide-binding regulatory proteins (G proteins). These processes play an essential role in the regulation of cardiac function by hormones and neurotransmitters.

Gap junctional channels

Gap junction channels provide an enclosed conduit for direct exchange of molecules *between* cells, with diameters large enough to accommodate metabolites and signalling molecules with high molecular weights. The complete structure is made up of two connexons, one from each of the two

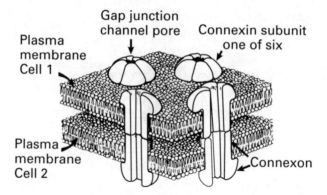

Figure 1.5 A gap junctional channel. (*From* Jongsma HJ, Rook MB. Morphology and electrophysiology of cardiac gap junction channels. In: Zipes D, Jalife J, eds. *Cardiac electrophysiology from cell to bedside*, 2nd edn. Philadelphia: WB Saunders, 1995.)

adjacent cells. Each connexon is composed of six connexin subunits, most likely arranged so that their third (out of four) transmembrane domains line the channel lumen (Figure 1.5). Complete gap junction channels are commonly clustered together and have extremely rapid turnover times, being exchanged several times a day. At least three types of connexin (C40, C43, C45) are expressed in the human heart.

Names and symbols for ionic currents

Although all cardiac ion channels share a common basic structure, there is undoubtedly a great variety of channels and corresponding currents in human cardiac myocytes. Although the function of all of these currents has yet to be identified, the majority make some contribution to the generation of either the resting or action potential (see Chapter 2). These currents can be influenced to varying degrees by abnormalities of ion channel function associated with genetic abnormalities, acquired insults such as ischaemia, and antiarrhythmic drug use.

All ion currents are described by the symbol I, together with a symbol for the appropriate ion, for example, I_{Na+}. The direction of the positive charge defines whether a transmembrane current is described as inward or outward, i.e. an inward current is one in which positively charged ions move into the cell. This results in the membrane potential becoming more positive (depolarisation). If positive ions move out of the cell this is referred to as hyperpolarisation. Current flow across an open ion channel is dependent upon the electromotive force (voltage or potential difference) generated by the ionic gradient across the membrane. The relationship between current flow and voltage may not be linear, in which case the channel is said to exhibit rectification. Rectification can be inward or outward depending on whether the conductance is higher in the outward or inward direction.

Descriptions of the major ion currents

Sodium current (I_{Na+})

This is the major inward current, depolarising cardiac cells in the atria, ventricles, and Purkinje fibres during phase 0 of the action potential (see Chapter 2). I_{Na+} is not thought to be involved in the action potentials of sinoatrial or atrioventricular nodes. A number of antiarrhythmic agents in common use have a reduction in I_{Na+} as their main mode of action (so called class I action, see Chapter 16).

Calcium currents

Calcium currents are of two types. *L-type* calcium current (I_{Ca-L}) (L for large and long lasting) is the dominant calcium current in all mature cardiac cells and (a) provides the sustained inward current that is partially responsible for the plateau phase (phase 2) of the action potential and (b) couples the electrical phenomenon of cell depolarisation to cardiac myocyte contraction. The *T-type* calcium current (I_{Ca-T}) (T for transient) is usually seen in atrial, Purkinje, and nodal cells whilst in ventricular cells it is of small amplitude and sometimes cannot be demonstrated, suggesting it is not vital to excitation contraction coupling. This current is a transient current elicited by small depolarisations above the resting potential level. It inactivates rapidly and, unlike I_{Ca-L}, is insensitive to dihydropyridines such as verapamil. The physiological role of I_{Ca-T} is most likely to be in pacemaker impulse generation given its clear demonstration in sinus node and AV nodal tissue.

Delayed rectifier potassium current (I_K)

The delayed rectifier potassium current I_K is an outward current important in the repolarisation of the cardiac action potential. It consists of I_{Kr}, a rapidly activating current with a sensitivity to the antiarrhythmic agent sotalol, and I_{Ks}, a slowly activating current.

Background potassium current (I_{K1})

The background potassium current is a reflection of the much higher concentration of K^+ ions within cardiac cells and the relatively high resting permeability of cardiac cells to potassium: this outward current is involved in setting the cell resting membrane potential (see Chapter 2). This current (also termed inward rectifier) is not usually present in nodal cells, and as a consequence the resting potentials of these cells are less negative than those of atrial, ventricular, and Purkinje cells.

Transient outward current (I_{TO})

I_{TO} is activated by the rapid depolarisation associated with I_{Na+} and is responsible for the transient repolarisation in phase 1 of the action potential.

I_{Kur}

This current is present in atrial cells only and, together with I_{TO}, is responsible for phase 1 of the action potential of the atria but not the ventricles.

$I_{K(ATP)}$

$I_{K(ATP)}$ is a current that is sensitive to cytosolic levels of ATP. In the presence of low ATP levels, such as during ischaemia, the current is activated, resulting in efflux of potassium and hyperpolarisation.

$I_{K(ACh)}$

$I_{K(ACh)}$ is a similar current to I_{K1} and is activated by the acetylcholine muscarinic receptor on the cell membrane. This receptor is coupled to the potassium channel via membrane-bound G protein. Activation by acetylcholine results in potassium efflux and hyperpolarisation of the cell associated with vagal stimulation.

Hyperpolarisation-activated current or pacemaker current (I_f)

The hyperpolarisation-activated current or pacemaker current I_f is one of the candidates for the generation of pacemaker activity in the sinus node. F is for "funny" because of the unusual properties of the current: sodium ions carry the charge through the channel and current activation starts at approximately 40 mV to -50 mV.

Background pumps

Cardiac cells have ion pumps that are important in the re-establishment of ion gradients following activity. The sodium potassium pump (3NA : 2K) causes an outward current because it pumps three sodium ions out for every two potassium ions in. Activity of this pump is reduced by digoxin, allowing accumulation of intracellular sodium. This then leads to intracellular accumulation of calcium (via a sodium/calcium exchanger mechanism) that is thought to be the basis for the positive inotropic and arrhythmogenic effects of this agent.

Non-specific calcium-activated current (I_{TI} or transient inward current)

This is an oscillatory membrane current carried by sodium ions that is triggered by a rise in cytoplasmic calcium concentrations. It is a mechanism of delayed after-depolarisations and sometimes early after-depolarisations (see Chapter 2).

Further reading

Catterall WA *et al.* Molecular bases of ion channel activity. In: Zipes D, Jalife J, eds. *Cardiac electrophysiology from cell to bedside*, 2nd edn. Philadelphia: WB Saunders, 1995.

Hodgkin AL, Huxley AF. A quantitative description of membrane current and its application to conduction and excitation in nerve. *J Physiol (Lond)* 1952;**117**:500–44.

Jalife J, Delmar M, Davidenko JM, Anumonwo JMB. *Basic cardiac electrophysiology for the clinician.* New York: Futura Publishing, 1999.

Noble D. *The initiation of the heart beat.* New York: Oxford University Press, 1979.

2: The cardiac action potential and its relevance to arrhythmias

Whilst it is frequently stated that understanding of the details of the cardiac action potential is (or will be) important for an understanding of cardiac arrhythmias in patients, it is not immediately obvious why this should be true. Most clinical cardiac arrhythmias are caused by abnormalities in propagation through tissues (see Chapter 3) rather than abnormalities in physiology of individual cells. Nevertheless, some clinical arrhythmias are undoubtedly explicable in terms of abnormalities in the action potential (via abnormalities in ion currents) and these will be discussed following a description of the normal action potential in cardiac cells.

The resting potential

In the majority of atrial and ventricular myocytes, the voltage across the cell membrane (resting potential) remains constant between action potentials at approximately -85 mV, a level which is primarily determined by the fact that the cell membrane in this state is much more permeable to potassium than to other ions. The membrane potential is the consequence of a balance between the chemical or concentration gradient for K^+ ions (high potassium inside, low potassium outside) pushing K^+ ions out of the cell (I_{K1}), leading to an opposing electrical gradient across the membrane consequent upon the removal of positive charge from the cell (Figure 2.1).

The action potential

The generation of the sustained depolarisation known as the action potential is the means whereby electrical impulses are transmitted rapidly through excitable tissues. The classic description of the cardiac action potential is based upon that of a Purkinje fibre, in which there are four distinct phases (Figure 2.2). Phase 0 is the rapid upstroke phase, phase 1 is the brief initial repolarisation phase, phase 2 is the plateau phase, phase 3 the rapid repolarisation phase, and phase 4 is the period between the end of one action potential and the beginning of the next, which in the Purkinje

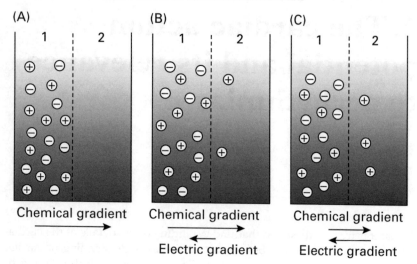

Figure 2.1 Origin of the resting potential. A vessel is divided into two compartments (1 and 2) by a membrane that is permeable to positive ions (potassium) but impermeable to negative ions. Placing an ionisable solution into compartment 1 creates a chemical concentration gradient for the flow of positive ions toward compartment 2(*A*). As positive ions move across the membrane, they leave negative ions behind, generating an electric gradient of direction opposite to the chemical one (*B*). Steady state is achieved when the magnitude of the chemical and electric gradients are equal (*C*). (*From* Jalife J, Delmar M, Davidenko JM, Anumonwo JMB. *Basic cardiac electrophysiology for the clinician.* Armonk, NY: Futura Publishing, 1999.)

fibre corresponds to the non-excited or resting potential. The action potential as described above can be considered an "all-or-nothing" phenomenon, i.e. once phase 0 has been triggered, the remaining phases automatically follow (time dependence).

Ionic changes associated with the action potential

The inward sodium current is activated once the membrane potential of a Purkinje fibre depolarises above a certain threshold value (threshold potential) (Figure 2.3). The concentration of Na^+ in the extracellular space is significantly greater than the intracellular space (140 mM v 4 mM) and once the Na^+ channels open there is a very large, rapid influx of positively charged Na^+ ions into the cell, resulting in phase 0 depolarisation. After a few milliseconds the Na^+ channels are inactivated and the depolarisation stops at approximately +20 mV. In most cardiac cells the phase 1 repolarisation is provided by the transient outward current (I_{TO}) of potassium ions which itself inactivates very rapidly. The dominant currents during the plateau phase of the action potential are the inward long-lasting calcium current (I_{Ca-L}) (maintaining depolarisation) and the delayed

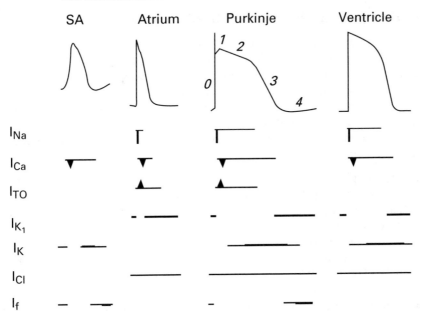

Figure 2.2   Phases of the action potential in a Purkinje fibre and differences in action potential morphology in myocytes from different parts of the heart. (*From* Hondeghem LM. Use dependence and reverse use dependence of antiarrhythmic agents: pro and antiarrhythmic actions. In: Breithardt G, Borggrefe M, Camm J, Shenasa M, eds. *Antiarrhythmic drugs*. Berlin: Springer, 1994.)

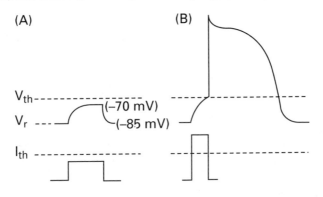

Figure 2.3   Generation of the action potential requires depolarisation of the membrane potential (by a current injection) above a certain threshold value (*B*). If this threshold is not reached (*A*) no action potential results. (*From* Jalife J, Delmar M, Davidenko JM, Anumonwo JMB. *Basic cardiac electrophysiology for the clinician.* New York: Futura, 1999.)

rectifier potassium outward current (I_K) (causing repolarisation). Phase 3 occurs when Ca^{2+} channels are inactivated and the outward potassium currents are unopposed. The delayed rectifier current inactivates as the cell repolarises, and finally I_{K1} predominates (phase 4).

13

Action potentials in specialised cardiac cells

The classic action potential as described above shows important variations depending upon exactly which cardiac cells are involved (see Figure 2.2). Perhaps the most important variation relates to the action potential of the sinus node, where normal cardiac electrical activity is initiated. *Sinus node cells*, unlike atrial or ventricular myocytes, spontaneously depolarise without any excitatory stimulus being required from another cell. This pacemaker activity is associated with two major differences in action potential characteristics from a "generic" myocyte.

- During phase 4 there is a slow spontaneous depolarisation that brings the membrane potential from its most negative point at the end of repolarisation (approximately $-60\,mV$ in sinus node cells) to the threshold potential at the onset of the next action potential (see Figure 2.2). Despite many years of research, the mechanisms responsible for this vital "pacemaker current" remain controversial. The most commonly held view is that it results from a hyperpolarisation-activated sodium current called I_f.

- The action potential upstroke of sinus nodal cells is slower than that of ventricular myocytes and starts at a more negative threshold potential. These characteristics are the result of the depolarisation being dependent on Ca^{2+} ions through channels similar to those mediating $I_{Ca^{2+}}$ in ventricular cells. The sodium current and inward rectifier potassium current (I_{K1}) are virtually absent from sinus node cells.

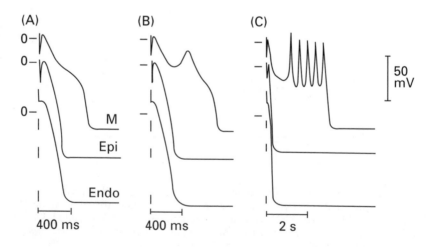

Figure 2.4   Quinidine-induced early after-depolarisations and triggered activity in an M cell. (*From* Antzelevitch C, Di Diego JM, Sicouri S and Lukas A. Selective pharmacological modification of repolarising currents: antiarrhythmic and proarrhythmic actions of agents that influence repolarisation in the heart. In: Breithardt G, Borggrefe M, Camm J, Shenasa M, eds. *Antiarrhythmic drugs.* Berlin: Springer, 1994.)

Atrioventricular nodal cells in the centre or N region of the AV node show action potentials similar to sinus node cells and indeed have intrinsic pacemaker properties, although spontaneous depolarisations are at a slower rate than those from the sinus node.

M cells are located in the middle myocardium (between the subendocardial and subepicardial regions) and have longer action potential durations than cells located in the other regions (Figure 2.4A).

Relevance of the action potential to clinical arrhythmias

Abnormalities of the action potential that have the potential to cause clinical cardiac arrhythmias have historically been classified into three broad groups.

Normal automaticity of a cardiac cell can cause tachycardias if the rate of spontaneous phase 4 depolarisation increases but such situations are very rarely pathological. The most common example is that of exercise-related sinus tachycardia in which phase 4 depolarisation of the sinus node is increased by sympathetic activation and vagal inhibition.

Abnormal automaticity has been described in isolated atrial or ventricular cells in which the resting potential has been made less negative than normal by some intervention such as ischaemia. This can result in spontaneous phase 4 depolarisations carried by Ca^{2+} ions (Figure 2.5). It has yet to be shown convincingly that such preparations have a clinical counterpart but animal studies have suggested that they may play a role in ventricular arrhythmias in the early period after myocardial infarction.

Triggered activity refers to depolarisations caused by oscillations in membrane potential that follow an action potential upstroke and are termed after-depolarisations (Figure 2.6). If such after-depolarisations occur during phases 2 or 3 they are referred to as early after-depolarisations (EADs), and if they are in phase 4, as delayed after-depolarisations (DADs).

Experimentally, there is a wide variety of agents and conditions that can give rise to EADs but in general they share the common feature of prolonging repolarisation. An EAD occurs when, for some reason, the balance of repolarising currents changes so that there is a net inward movement of charge. This can occur as a consequence of a decrease in outward potassium

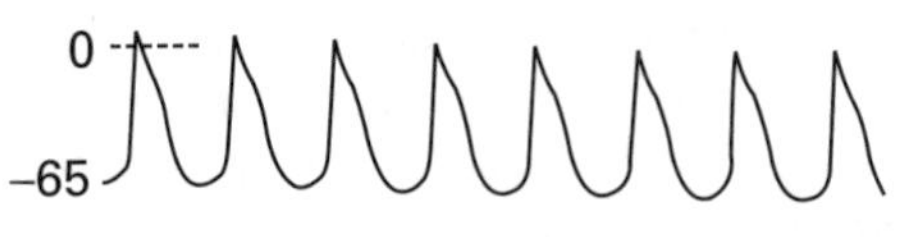

Figure 2.5   Action potentials from isolated Purkinje fibres in the endocardial border zone of a 24 hr old canine infarct, demonstrating spontaneous phase 4 depolarisations (abnormal automaticity). Heart rate is 140 bpm. (*From* Janse MM. *Mechanisms of arrhythmias.* New York: Futura, 1994.)

15

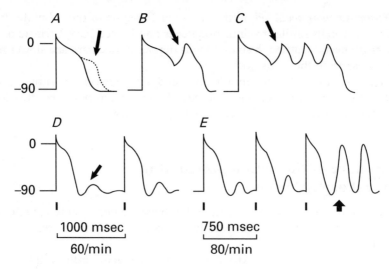

Figure 2.6 The development of triggered activity in association with early and later after-depolarisations. The solid trace in panel *A* shows the normal action potential of a Purkinje fibre. The dashed trace and arrow show the change in membrane potential during an early after-depolarisation. In panel *B* the arrow shows a second upstroke during phase 3 which was triggered by an early after-depolarisation. Panel *C* shows the second upstroke and two additional triggered impulses. In panel *D* a delayed after-depolarisation is indicated by the arrow. Delayed after-depolarisation amplitude increases when the stimulus rate is increased, as shown in panel *E*. Triggered activity occurs at the arrow when the after-depolarisation reaches threshold potential. (*From* Wit AL, Rosen MR. Cellular electrophysiology of cardiac arrhythmias. *Modern concepts of cardiovascular disease*. 1981:**50** 7–11.)

current or an increase in the inward sodium or calcium currents. EADs occur more readily in Purkinje fibres than in ventricular or atrial muscle. However, the M cell located in the deep subepicardium and midmyocardium is prone to the development of EADs (Figure 2.4). They may well play a role in in the long QT syndrome (see Chapter 12), in which ventricular arrhythmias are associated with prolongation of the QT interval on the surface electrocardiogram.

Delayed after-depolarisations (DADs) occur in experimental preparations of cellular Ca^{2+} overload and are thought to be implicated in arrhythmias associated with digoxin toxicity. Calcium overload, from whatever cause, results in a transient inward sodium current (I_{TI}) through a calcium-dependent non-specific ion channel, giving rise to a DAD. Exogenously administered adenosine has been used as a specific test for the diagnosis of tachycardias dependent upon DADs. Adenosine reduces I_{ca} indirectly by inhibiting adenylate cyclase and cAMP. Adenosine terminates and suppresses right ventricular outflow tract tachycardia suggesting that the mechanism of this arrhythmia is cAMP-mediated triggered activity (see Chapter 8).

Further reading

Hoffman BF, Rosen MR. Cellular mechanisms for cardiac arrhythmias. *Circ Res* 1981;**49**:1–15.

Jalife J, Delmar M, Davidenko JM, Anumonwo JMB. *Basic cardiac electrophysiology for the clinician*. New York: Futura Publishing, 1999.

Lerman BB, Belardinelli L, West GA *et al*. Adenosine-sensitive ventricular tachycardia: evidence suggesting cyclic AMP-mediated triggered activity. *Circulation* 1986;**74**:270–280.

Noble D. *The initiation of the heart beat*. New York: Oxford University Press, 1979.

3: Propagation of electrical impulses through cardiac muscle

Whilst much attention has been directed at the electrical events involved in excitation of single cardiac cells, in terms of the generation of clinical tachycardias it is likely that the mechanisms of propagation of the cardiac impulse *between* cells are just as important (or perhaps more so).

Local current spread (electrotonic propagation)

Injection of current across the membrane of a single myocyte will not only lead to the depolarisation of the membrane of that particular cell but will also lead to propagation of excitation across the intercellular gap junctions to the neighbouring cells. The voltage change that results from such a current injection is described by the "cable equations" originally devised to characterise changes in a transatlantic telegraphic cable. They describe the changes in voltage along a continuous passive fibre in which resistance is constant throughout. When a current pulse is introduced into such a fibre the amplitude of the resulting depolarisation decays exponentially with distance (Figure 3.1). This form of propagation of cellular excitation occurs in the absence of generation of action potentials and describes the behaviour of cell membrane below threshold levels (electrotonic propagation). The diameter of the fibre has a major influence on the cable type properties, with intracellular resistances increasing as fibre diameter is reduced. In other words, the length of the fibre that is influenced locally by a given current pulse from a point source is greater in a thick than a thin fibre.

There are limitations to the use of cable equations in that propagation along cardiac tissue is not perfectly uniform and there are microscopic discontinuities in the form of gap junctions. Nevertheless, under normal circumstances the small delays imposed by the gap junctions are of relatively minor significance.

Propagation of the action potential

It can be seen from the above that the electrotonic form of propagation through cardiac muscle is unlikely to be an effective means of rapid spread

18

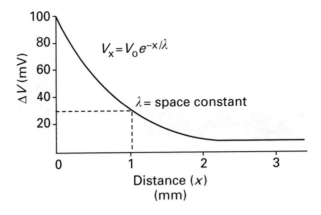

Figure 3.1 The exponential decay of potential difference across the cell membrane with distance. (*From* Jalife J, Delmar M, Davidenko JM, Anumonwo JMB. *Basic cardiac electrophysiology for the clinician.* Armonk, NY: Futura, 1999.)

of electrical activity throughout the heart because of the rapid fall in voltage with distance along the muscle fibre. Co-ordinated activation of the heart is made possible by the generation of action potentials, the all or nothing nature of which provides a "boost" for the propagating impulse as each cell is reached, thereby ensuring there is no decay of voltage with distance. The depolarisation current generated by the first action potential propagates electrotonically to the next cell which then reaches its threshold potential and a second action potential occurs with a new influx of inward current which becomes the source of current for cells further downstream. In a linear cable composed of electrically interconnected excitable cells, impulse propagation is determined primarily by the ratio between the current available to excite cells (the source) and the current required by cells downstream to be excited (referred to as the sink), i.e. the likelihood of successful propagation (sometimes termed safety factor for conduction) from proximal to distal cells in such a cable is proportional to the excess of source current over the requirement of the distal cells that form the sink. Slow conduction and/or conduction block may result from a progressive decrease in this ratio or safety factor.

The current generated by the proximal part of the cable (source) is determined by:

- The maximum rate of rise of the action potential upstroke
- Action potential amplitude
- Action potential duration.

Antiarrhythmic drugs may cause conduction slowing or conduction block by reducing any of these factors (see Chapter 16).

Passive membrane properties related to cell-to-cell communication may also modulate the amount of excitatory current delivered by the source. Perhaps less intuitively obvious is the influence of the sink. If the distal

19

(A)

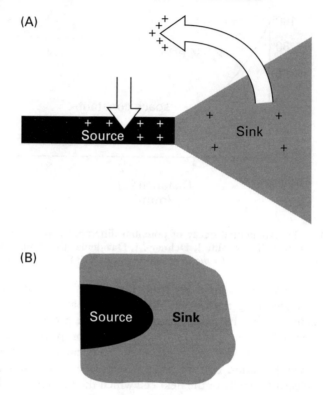

(B)

Figure 3.2   If a small group of myocytes acts as a source for current spread to a significantly greater number of distal cells, the source may be insufficient to depolarise the "sink" and the impulse may slow or fail to propagate. If a proximal group of cells activates distal cells over a broad area (as in the case of a curved wave front) conduction slowing and failure of propagation is more likely than if the source acts as a planar wave. (*From* Jalife J, Delmar M, Davidenko JM, Anumonwo JMB. *Basic cardiac electrophysiology for the clinician.* Armonk, NY: Futura, 1999.)

myocytes being activated are in a two-dimensional sheet (or a three-dimensional block) rather than behaving as a single cable, there may come a point during propagation of an action potential when a single myocyte or a small group of myocytes must act as the source for current spread to a significantly greater number of distal cells (Figure 3.2A). This situation may occur when a thin unbranched uniform array of cardiac cells exists in the middle of infarcted ventricular muscle connected to a broad sheet of healthy ventricular myocytes on the edge of the infarcted area. Under these circumstances the source may provide insufficient current to depolarise the broad sheet of distal cells and the impulse may fail to propagate. In other words, there is a "loading effect" imposed by the cells downstream on a proximal source. In this way the geometry of cardiac muscle fibres can greatly influence the likelihood of successful propagation of the cardiac impulse throughout the heart.

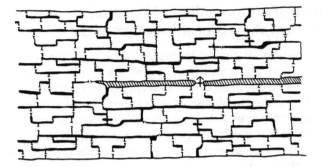

Figure 3.3   Structure of cardiac muscle showing a schematic drawing of two adjacent "unit bundles" of cardiac muscle cells and their interconnections. It can be seen that the myocardium is better coupled in the direction of the long axis of its cells and bundles (anisotropy), because of the architecture of the myocytes and positioning of the gap junctions. (*From* Sommer JR and Dolber PC. Cardiac muscle: ultrastructure of its cells and bundles. In Paes de Carvalho A, Hoffman BF, Lieberman M, eds. *Normal and abnormal conduction in the heart*. Mt Kisco, NY: Futura, 1982.)

Anisotropic propagation

One of the fundamental characteristics of electrical propagation through cardiac tissue is that it is directionally dependent: this is the consequence of the rod-like shape of adult cardiac myocytes, the heterogeneous distribution of gap junctions and the orientation of cell bundles along the long axis of the cells (Figure 3.3). As a consequence, speed of propagation is three to five times greater in the longitudinal direction (parallel to fibre direction) than the transverse direction. This directional dependence of propagation is referred to as anisotropy. Although conduction velocity is greater in the longitudinal direction, the directional dependence of the safety factor for conduction may be greater in the longitudinal or transverse direction depending upon, amongst other factors, relative resistivity in the two directions. Asymmetry in the safety factor for conduction may result in conduction block occurring in one particular direction (unidirectional block) and this is likely to be important in the generation of cardiac arrhythmias (see later).

Propagation of curved wave fronts

It follows from the discussion of the influence of a distal sheet of cells on propagation velocity and safety factor for conduction that the shape of a propagated wave front is a major determinant of success or failure of propagation. It is clear that the relative area of distal tissue to be excited (the sink) ahead of a convexly curved wave front (the source) is larger than the area forming the sink in front of an equivalent plane wave (Figure 3.2B). The more convexly curved a wave front, the lower its velocity of propagation and the higher the likelihood of failure of conduction.

21

Relevance of abnormalities in propagation to cardiac arrhythmias: the generation of re-entry

The great majority of clinical tachycardias have a re-entrant mechanism, i.e. are caused by abnormalities in propagation of the electrical impulse through cardiac tissue rather than abnormalities in activation of individual cells. Re-entry is the circulation of the cardiac impulse around an obstacle (anatomical or functional) leading to repetitive excitation at a frequency that depends on the conduction velocity of the impulse and the perimeter of the obstacle. There are three principal requirements for re-entrant activity to occur (Figure 3.4).

- The presence of a circuit which can be either anatomically or functionally determined. The classic example of an anatomic re-entrant circuit

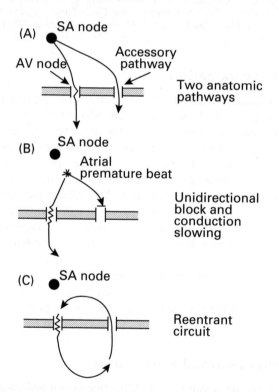

Figure 3.4 Requirements for re-entrant activity as demonstrated in the anatomic re-entrant circuit associated with the Wolff–Parkinson–White syndrome. (A) The existence of two potential routes for electrical wave fronts (in this case the AV node and accessory pathway). (B) An atrial premature beat finds one route refractory (the accessory pathway), leading to unidirectional block in the accessory pathway. The prematurity of the atrial beat also leads to conduction slowing within the AV nodal tissue. (C) By the time the impulse reaches the ventricular end of the accessory pathway it is no longer refractory and a stable re-entrant circuit is formed.

is that associated with the Wolff–Parkinson–White syndrome (see Chapter 7), in which a clear and fixed anatomic abnormality exists. The circuit may be considered functionally determined if there is no well-defined anatomic circuit but a wave front circulates round a region of cardiac tissue that is inexcitable (or at least unexcited) in certain circumstances. The functional group of mechanisms probably underlies re-entrant activity associated with atrial and ventricular fibrillation.

- The need for unidirectional block for the initiation of circulating activity. This may occur as a consequence of a disparity in either refractoriness or safety factor for conduction between the two arms of the re-entrant circuit.
- The presence of slow conduction in some part of the circuit.

Anatomic re-entry

It is clear that for stable re-entrant activity to occur the rotation time around the circuit should be longer than the time required for recovery (termed refractory period) of any segment of the circuit. In other words, the wave length of refractoriness, which is the product of the refractory period and the conduction velocity, must be shorter than the perimeter of the circuit. Under these circumstances, an excitable gap will appear between the head of the circulating impulse and its own refractory tail (Figure 3.5A). The shorter the wave length (due to either short refractoriness and/or slow conduction velocities), the larger the excitable gap, and the more stable the re-entrant tachycardia. Re-entrant activity will be stable in the presence of a large excitable gap because the re-entrant wave front will find only fully recovered tissue in its path. Tissue that is partially recovered may be excitable but may also lead to failure of propagation.

As will be discussed in later chapters, anatomic re-entry is responsible for many clinical tachycardias, including atrial flutter, AV nodal re-entrant tachycardia, tachycardias associated with the Wolff–Parkinson–White syndrome and several forms of ventricular tachycardia.

Functional re-entry

Functional re-entry occurs in the absence of a predetermined structural circuit.

The leading circle model of functional re-entry

According to the leading circle concept, a propagated wave turns back on its own refractory "tail" and re-entrant activity occurs: (1) without an excitable gap and (2) with a size that is determined by refractoriness of the cardiac tissue (Figure 3.5B). It is postulated that the central core of tissue around which the impulse propagates remains inexcitable because it is continually being depolarised electronically by the circulating wave and therefore continually refractory.

23

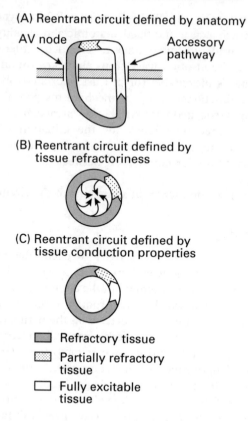

Figure 3.5   Different forms of re-entry.

(*A*) Re-entrant circuit defined by anatomy: in this example orthodromic tachycardia associated with an accessory pathway. In this situation the size of the re-entrant circuit is defined by anatomic boundaries. At any particular moment a length of the electrical tissue within the circuit is completely refractory (the wavelength of refractoriness, defined as refractory period × conduction velocity). A further length will be partially refractory and the remaining length remains available for excitation (excitable gap). The larger the excitable gap the less likely that the advancing wave front will encounter refractory tissue and the more stable the re-entrant circuit.

(*B*) Re-entrant circuit defined by tissue refractoriness. In the leading circle model of functional re-entry an advancing wave front rotates back upon itself, the diameter of the rotating circuit being limited only by the wavelength of refractoriness (*see above*). In this model there is no excitable gap and the core of the wavelet is rendered continuously refractory by continuous re-excitation from the surrounding circulating electrical activity.

(*C*) Re-entrant circuit defined by tissue conduction properties. In this form of functional re-entry (spiral wave hypothesis) the size of the re-entrant circuit is determined by the ability of the wave front to curve back upon itself. In contrast to the leading circle model of functional re-entry, in this scheme an excitable gap may exist and the core remains available for excitation.

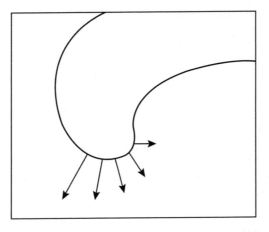

Figure 3.6   Wavefront curvature is highest at the centre of a spiral wave and as a consequence conduction is slowest at this point. (*From* Jalife J, Delmar M, Davidenko JM, Anumonwo JMB. *Basic cardiac electrophysiology for the clinician.* Armonk, NY: Futura, 1999.)

Spiral waves

Some authors have suggested that the properties of functional re-entrant waves are governed mainly by the properties of curved wave fronts rather than the leading circle explanation discussed above. It is suggested that the formation of rotating spiral waves is a common feature of excitable tissues throughout biology and that their formation is related to the effect of curvature on propagating wave fronts. It can be seen that, during spiral wave activity, curvature of the wave front is extremely high at the centre of the spiral and it is proposed that (due to source/sink mismatch) it is sufficiently high to result in failure of propagation (Figure 3.6): thus the dynamics of propagation of curved wave fronts may explain the origin of this core. A consequence of the above hypothesis is that, as opposed to the leading circle mechanism, an excitable gap may well be present during these rotating waves (Figure 3.5C), and indeed this can be demonstrated directly by the fact that externally induced propagating waves with lower curvature (and therefore higher speed) are able to invade the core region during spiral wave activity. Because the core remains excitable during spiral wave activity, it is not surprising that small changes in the condition of the spiral wave tip (such as small changes in the excitability of the tissue) may lead to shifts in the trajectory of the spiral wave, leading to "drifting spirals". This is currently a popular hypothesis for the mechanism of atrial and ventricular fibrillation.

Anisotropic re-entry

Anisotropic re-entry may be considered as a form of functionally determined re-entry in which initiation and maintenance of the re-entrant activity is based on the directional properties of the tissue. As has been discussed previously, propagation velocity in cardiac muscle is three to five times faster in the longitudinal axis of the cells than along the transverse axis. Similarly, there is asymmetry in the safety factor for propagation as well as conduction velocity. Thus, anisotropy may set the stage for heterogeneity of functional properties and unidirectional block and lead to the initiation and maintenance of re-entry. Clear clinical examples of such forms of re-entry are difficult to come across, however. It has been suggested, based on a dog model of ventricular tachycardia following myocardial infarction, that anisotropic propagation may play a major role in the initiation and maintenance of re-entry in ventricular tissue surviving a myocardial infarction.

Further reading

Danse PW, Garratt CJ, Allessie MA. Preferential depression of conduction around a pivot point in rabbit ventricular myocardium by potassium and flecainide. *J Cardiovasc Electrophysiol* 2000;**11**:262–273.

El-Sherif N. Re-entrant mechanisms in ventricular arrhythmias. In: Zipes D and Jalife J eds. *Cardiac electrophysiology from cell to bedside*, 2nd edn. Philadelphia: WB Saunders, 1995.

Fast VG, Kleber AG. Role of wavefront curvature in propagation of the cardiac impulse. *Cardiovasc Res* 1997;**33**:258–271.

Jalife J, Delmar M, Davidenko JM, Anumonwo JMB. *Basic cardiac electrophysiology for the clinician*. New York: Futura Publishing, 1999.

PART II
CLINICAL TACHYCARDIAS

4: Classification and nomenclature of clinical tachycardias

Tachycardias are usually classified according to their presumed site of origin. It is obvious that, as knowledge about the site of origin of tachycardias has increased, so the terms used to describe arrhythmias have become more specific. It is usual to classify arrhythmias into three broad groups based on whether they originate in the atrium, the atrioventricular junction, or the ventricle. The following description is not an exhaustive list, but includes all the common tachycardias and all those discussed in this book. This classification acts as a framework for the subsequent chapters and includes some terms that will be fully defined and described in the relevant section.

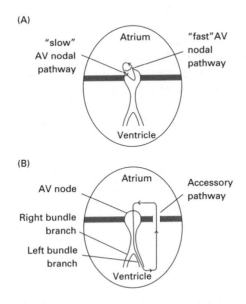

Figure 4.1   Anatomic basis for the two common forms of junctional tachycardia: atrioventricular nodal re-entrant tachycardia (*A*) and atrioventricular re-entrant tachycardia utilising an accessory pathway (*B*).

Tachycardias originating in the atrium

- Sinus tachycardia
- Atrial tachycardia
- Atrial flutter
- Atrial fibrillation.

Tachycardias originating in the atrioventricular junction (Figure 4.1)

- Atrioventricular nodal re-entrant tachycardia (AVNRT)
- Accessory pathway mediated re-entrant tachycardia (sometimes referred to as atrioventricular re-entrant tachycardia or AVRT)

Prior to the full description of the source of these tachycardias they were often referred to as PAT (paroxysmal atrial tachycardia) or PSVT (paroxysmal supraventricular tachycardia). When the precise diagnosis is unclear but thought to be either AVNRT or AVRT, then the phrase paroxysmal junctional tachycardia is appropriate.

Tachycardias originating in the ventricle

Subclassification of ventricular arrhythmias is based primarily on their electrocardiographic morphology (Figure 4.2):

- Monomorphic ventricular tachycardia (including right ventricular outflow tract tachycardia, left ventricular fascicular tachycardia)
- Polymorphic ventricular tachycardia (sometimes referred to as torsade de pointes, when there is a typical "twisting of the points" appearance or (more loosely) if polymorphic ventricular tachycardia occurs in the setting of a long QT interval
- Ventricular fibrillation (polymorphic ventricular tachycardia that is associated with cessation of cardiac output and does not self-terminate)
- Ventricular flutter – very rapid monomorphic ventricular tachycardia (usually 300 beats/min or more) that is associated with cessation of cardiac output.

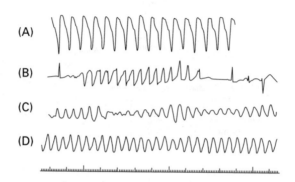

Figure 4.2   Monomorphic ventricular tachycardia (A), polymorphic ventricular tachycardia (B), ventricular fibrillation (C), and ventricular flutter (D).

5: Sinus tachycardia, atrial tachycardia, and atrial flutter

Sinus tachycardia

Sinus tachycardia is the normal physiological response to a number of stimuli, including exercise, anxiety, fever, pain, hypotension, pulmonary embolism, and other acute medical conditions. The key electrocardiographic feature of sinus tachycardia is the presence of P waves of normal morphology during tachycardia (Figure 5.1). Under these circumstances it is not appropriate to attempt to slow the heart rate, as the tachycardia may be the only thing maintaining an adequate circulation. The cause of the tachycardia should be sought and treatment directed appropriately.

There are two conditions in which sinus tachycardia is not a normal physiological or compensatory response. *Sinus node re-entrant tachycardia* (SNRT), as the name implies, is a re-entrant tachycardia in which the circuit involves the sinus node or perinodal tissue, and may represent a specific form of focal atrial tachycardia (see below). It differs from other forms of sinus tachycardia in that it has a sudden (within one beat) onset and offset. P wave morphology is, by definition, normal. Patients rarely present with this tachycardia and much more frequently it is a coincidental finding at electrophysiology study. Treatment is rarely necessary but beta blockade or verapamil are usually effective.

Inappropriate sinus tachycardia usually occurs in young people, predominantly women, and may be an expression of what is known as the hyperadrenergic syndrome. In this syndrome the presentation is with troublesome palpitation that may be present throughout most of the day. Attempts to record cardiac rhythm coincident with symptoms reveals sinus tachycardia only, usually in the 110–140 beats per minute range. This syndrome overlaps with orthostatic intolerance syndrome, which is characterised by symptoms of lightheadedness and fatigue in addition to palpitations and is associated with a marked rise in heart rate on standing. This syndrome in turn overlaps with the chronic fatigue syndrome. It has been suggested that the hyperadrenergic syndromes are an expression of oversensitivity of the heart to circulating catecholamines, and certainly these patients have a particularly high heart rate in response to intravenous catecholamine infusion.

31

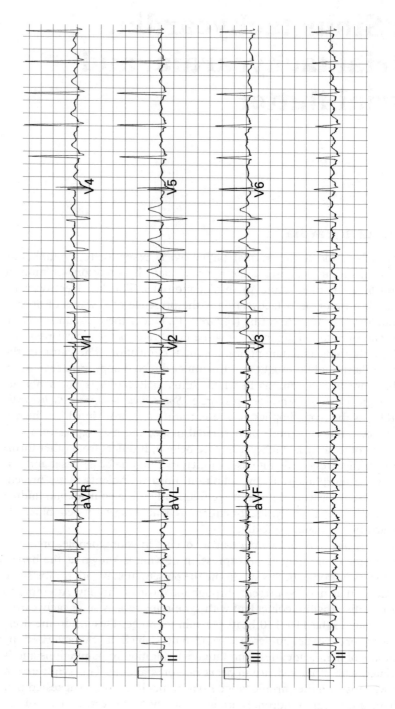

Figure 5.1 12-lead ECG of sinus tachycardia. Normal P waves can clearly be seen preceding the QRS complexes.

Beta blockade should be attempted in the first instance, but these patients are usually poorly tolerant of this and other medication. As a result, these patients commonly progress from one medication to another (and often one doctor to another) with little improvement.

Attempts to modify the sinus node in cases of inappropriate sinus tachycardia have shown that extensive radiofrequency applications must be performed in order to accomplish a moderate sinus rate reduction. There is a high recurrence rate and such a procedure is certainly one of last resort. Patients must understand that only those symptoms clearly associated with a rapid heart rate can improve with sinus node ablation.

Atrial tachycardias

Atrial tachycardias are defined as supraventricular arrhythmias that require atrial tissue only (i.e. not AV junctional or ventricular tissue) for initiation and maintenance. A variety of features have been used to classify these arrhythmias, such as the putative cellular mechanism, features of the surface electrocardiogram, response to drugs and the presence or absence of prior cardiac surgery. For instance, atrial tachycardias that can be terminated by intravenous adenosine are thought to have an automatic mechanism, whereas those that can reproducibly be initiated or terminated by atrial premature beats are thought to have a re-entrant mechanism. Increasingly, however, they are classified with catheter ablation techniques in mind and can be subdivided as follows.

Tachycardias that arise from a focal area of atrial tissue

These tachycardias can be cured by delivery of radiofrequency application at a specific site. The most common atrial sites which can give rise to such arrhythmias are the terminal crest (crista terminalis) in the right atrium, the junction of the left atrium with the pulmonary veins, and the junction of the superior caval vein with the right atrium (Figure 5.2). It is unclear why such sites are particularly important in the generation of atrial tachycardia, but it may be that local discontinuities of atrial structure are important in the generation of micro re-entry. Alternatively such sites may be more susceptible to stretch-induced abnormal automaticity.

Although a likely cellular mechanism (re-entry, automaticity, or triggered activity) may be delineated in some cases, successful application of radiofrequency energy (and cure) is independent of the suggested cellular mechanism.

Clinical and electrocardiographic presentation

The clinical settings in which this type of atrial tachycardia occur are very much those of atrial flutter and atrial fibrillation (see Chapter 6). Clinical presentation is usually with palpitations but may be with symptoms associated with a tachycardia-induced cardiomyopathy. P wave morphology is abnormal (unlike sinus tachycardia) and gives a good indication of the site

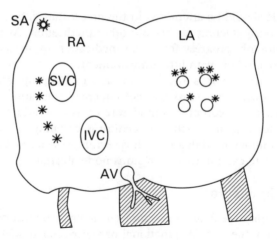

Figure 5.2   Schematic representation of usual sites of focal atrial tachycardias: the terminal crest in the right atrium and at the junction with the pulmonary veins in the left atrium.

of origin of the tachycardia (Figure 15.2). Positive P waves in the inferior leads indicate a superior (rather than inferior) origin and a positive P wave in V1 indicates a left atrial origin. Rarely, P wave morphology may be variable ("multifocal" atrial tachycardia), particularly if it is occurring in the setting of illnesses associated with elevated right-sided intracardiac pressures such as acute exacerbations of pulmonary disease.

Therapy

Pharmacological treatment of patients with focal atrial tachycardias has been somewhat disappointing, and there are no controlled trials of medical therapy for these arrhythmias. Digoxin is frequently used in order to control the ventricular rate but does not affect the atrial tachycardia itself. Drugs such as flecainide and propafenone have been found to have efficacy rates of approximately 50% and amiodarone has also been shown to be moderately effective in terms of terminating and suppressing these arrhythmias. As with many other arrhythmias, recent attention has shifted to the role of radiofrequency catheter ablation as a curative treatment. Identification of the precise site of tachycardia origin (and therefore appropriate site for ablation lesions) at electrophysiology study is in general more difficult than for junctional tachycardias as sites are not limited to one anatomic structure, such as the AV junction. Reported success rates are in the order of 80–100% but recurrence may occur if there is widespread underlying atrial disease.

Tachycardias that involve re-entry with macroscopic anatomic and/or surgical barriers

In this category the critical re-entrant circuit involves (and is dependent upon) a region of atrial tissue (isthmus) that is delineated by anatomic

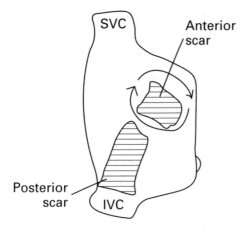

Figure 5.3   Representation of the re-entrant circuit in a patient with atriotomy-related atrial tachycardia, in this instance following repair of atrial septal defect. The presence of slowly conducting tissue between "islands" of non-conducting scar tissue predisposes to re-entrant arrhythmias. (*Modified from* Nakagawa *et al.* Characterisation of re-entrant circuit in macro re-entrant right atrial tachycardia after surgical repair of congenital heart disease. *Circulation* 2001; **103**:699–709.)

boundaries such as surgical atriotomy scars (Figure 5.3). Such "incisional" re-entrant atrial tachycardias involve a combination of natural and surgically created (incisions, patches, conduit material) barriers in patients following reparative surgery for congenital heart disease. In this situation a line (series of individual lesions) of radiofrequency lesions across the conducting isthmus is required to abolish the arrhythmia.

Clinical and electrocardiographic presentation

These arrhythmias can complicate repair of atrial septal defect, transposition of the great arteries (Mustard, Senning and Rastelli procedures) and Fontan procedures for tricuspid atresia, double inlet single ventricle, or other more complex anomalies. Incisional atrial tachycardias are usually sustained and may present several years after surgery. Usually the arrhythmias are of sudden onset and offset, and the electrocardiogram reveals a constant atrial cycle length of more than 0.2 seconds with an abnormal P wave morphology.

Therapy

The successful management of arrhythmias in these patients can be very challenging. As with the "focal" forms of atrial tachycardia, antiarrhythmic drugs are frequently ineffective. In addition, antiarrhythmic agents have the potential to adversely affect myocardial function and exacerbate coexisting sinus node dysfunction in such patients. Radiofrequency catheter ablation (as discussed above) is potentially curative in many such arrhythmias but requires a very high level of expertise in terms of mapping of the tachycardia circuit, identification of a critical isthmus and delivery of an uninterrupted line of lesions across this isthmus. Clinical reports in the literature indicate an acute success rate of 75–100% in terms of termination of these arrhythmias during ablation procedures, but there is a relatively high recurrence rate and overall success is probably not as high as that for junctional tachycardias (see Chapter 7). In severely symptomatic patients with tachycardia-induced cardiomyopathy (or the potential for this condition as indicated by an incessant arrhythmia with a rapid ventricular rate), radiofrequency ablation of the AV junction and pacemaker implantation may be considered. This may be a considerable challenge itself, depending upon the complexity of the underlying anatomy.

Atrial flutter

Atrial flutter was first described in 1911 and is a common arrhythmia that occurs in settings (and has the same causes) similar to atrial fibrillation (see following chapter). The two arrhythmias often coexist in the same patients.

Clinical presentation

Atrial flutter, like atrial fibrillation, can present in a paroxysmal or chronic form. Its most common presentation is a fast regular tachycardia with a ventricular rate of 150 beats per minute, representing an atrial rate of 300 beats/min conducted with 2:1 AV block (Figure 5.4). In situations in which AV nodal conduction is enhanced (for instance by high catecholamine drive or vagal withdrawal) or the flutter rate is slowed (usually by antiarrhythmic drugs), AV conduction may become 1:1 with associated marked haemodynamic deterioration (Figure 5.5). In addition to palpitations, patients may present with left ventricular dysfunction secondary to prolonged periods (weeks and months) of rapid ventricular rates, i.e. tachycardia-related cardiomyopathy.

Mechanism

"Typical" atrial flutter results from a large anatomic re-entrant circuit within the right atrium with the impulse travelling in a caudo-cranial direction up the interatrial septum and a cranio-caudal direction down the right free wall adjacent to the tricuspid annulus (referred to as a counterclockwise atrial flutter) (Figure 5.6). The tricuspid valve ring forms the anterior anatomic barrier of the circuit and a combination of the terminal crest and the eustachian ridge (between the inferior vena cava and the coronary sinus os) form the posterior anatomical barrier. More rarely, electrical activity travels in the reverse direction (counterclockwise) (Figure 5.7). An area of slow conduction is present in the muscular "isthmus" between the tricuspid valve ring and the inferior vena cava: this undoubtedly contributes to the stability of the anatomic re-entrant circuit (see Chapter 3) but is unlikely to be the primary abnormality as the electrophysiological characteristics of this area are similar in people without atrial flutter. It is more

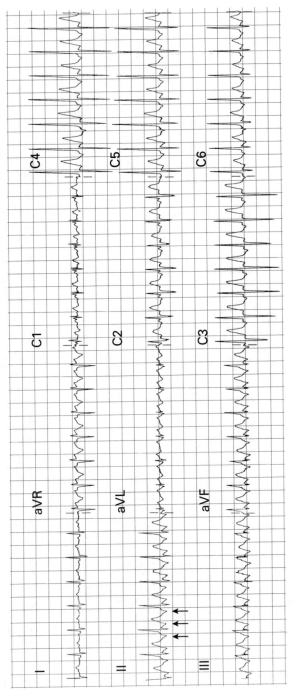

Figure 5.4 12-lead ECG of typical atrial flutter with 2:1 block: the characteristic negative flutter waves in the inferior leads are arrowed.

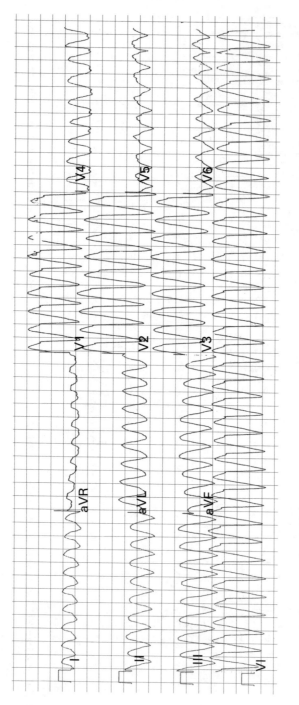

Figure 5.5 12-lead ECG of atrial flutter with 1:1 A:V conduction, producing a wide complex regular tachycardia with LBBB morphology. The atrial rate is slower than usual as the patient was taking flecainide. The diagnosis cannot be made purely on the basis of this ECG and the flecainide contributes to the widening of the QRS complex producing a VT-like appearance. Atrial flutter was suspected on the basis of previous atrial flutter with 2:1 block (in the absence of flecainide) and was confirmed by administration of adenosine.

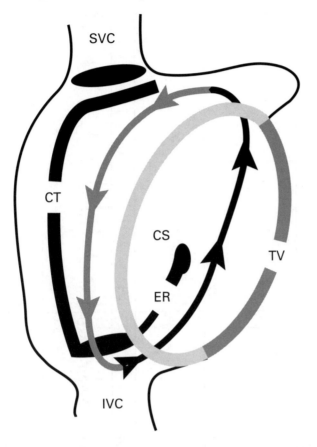

Figure 5.6 Schematic figure depicting the atrial flutter circuit rotating counter-clockwise around the tricuspid annulus. Note that the terminal crest (TC) and eustachian ridge (ER) act as lines of block preventing activation from "short circuiting" the annulus. (*Modified after* Olgin JE and Lesh MD. Role of anatomic structures and barriers in the ablation of atrial tachycardia and flutter. In: Huang S, Wilber D, eds. *Radiofrequency cathether ablation of cardiac arrhythmias.* Armonk, NY: Futura 2000.)

likely that the re-entrant activity develops because of an area of poor conduction within the atrial myocardium at the "centre" of the circuit, i.e. conduction across this region in normal people prevents the creation of a large re-entrant circuit encompassing a large part of the right atrium. The macro re-entrant nature of atrial flutter makes it very susceptible to catheter ablation techniques (see below).

Faster "type II" forms of atrial flutter involve smaller, less stable re-entrant circuits that are more likely to degenerate into atrial fibrillation and are not susceptible to catheter ablation. These circuits may not involve the tricuspid annulus/inferior vena cava isthmus and in many cases may not be anatomically fixed, i.e. have properties in common with atrial fibrillation.

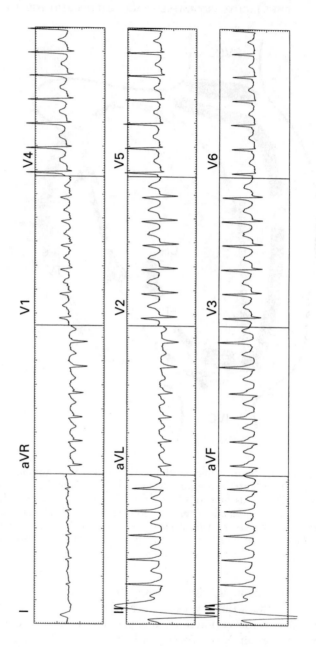

Figure 5.7   12-lead ECG of reverse typical atrial flutter.

Diagnosis

The presence of saw-toothed flutter waves in the ECG, particularly in lead II, remains the standard for the diagnosis of typical atrial flutter (see Figure 5.4).

Prognosis

It is increasingly recognised that the prognosis of atrial flutter is very similar to that of atrial fibrillation, although the latter arrhythmia has been studied in much greater detail. Risk of systemic embolism is thought to be significantly increased in those patients over 65 years of age, and those with structural heart disease or significant hypertension (see Chapter 6). Such patients should be anticoagulated if there is no identifiable contraindication.

Therapy

Pharmacological treatments for atrial flutter are usually disappointing. This may be related to the high level of stability in the re-entrant circuit conferred by the presence of a large excitable gap, which in turn is due to the large dimensions of the circuit. Agents that increase refractoriness (for example, potassium-channel blockers) are effective in at most 40–50% of cases. Agents that slow conduction (for example, flecainide) in general cause a slowing of the rate of the flutter waves rather than termination of the arrhythmia. This can lead to an increase in likelihood of 1:1 atrioventricular conduction during tachycardia and haemodynamic deterioration (see Figure 5.5). In the past, continuation of atrial flutter was accepted in many patients and the mainstay of pharmacological treatment was digoxin

Atrial flutter ablation

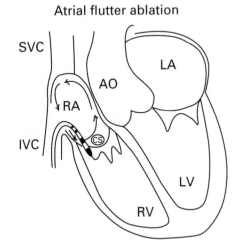

Figure 5.8 Schematic representation of initial catheter position for ablation of typical atrial flutter. RF energy is applied initially at the ventricular side of the tricuspid annulus caudal to the coronary sinus os and is then dragged back to the inferior vena cava, creating a continuous ablation line across the tricuspid isthmus.

to control the ventricular rate. The most effective methods of acutely terminating atrial flutter are DC cardioversion or rapid atrial pacing, in keeping with the re-entrant mechanism. If atrial pacing is employed, the atrial rate is increased to just above the flutter rate, allowing "capture" of the atrium from the pacemaker whilst minimising the risk of pacing-induced atrial fibrillation. High rate atrial pacing is usually required for a considerable time (15–30 seconds) before termination of tachycardia occurs and the pacing can be stopped. The success of pacing techniques is presumably related to the large excitable period during which paced beats can interrupt the re-entrant circuit. DC cardioversion is nearly always effective in the termination of atrial flutter and lower energies (for example, 100 J) are required than those usually necessary for the cardioversion of atrial fibrillation.

In recent years catheter ablation techniques have become the mainstay of curative treatment of recurrent or chronic atrial flutter. A line of ablation lesions is delivered over the slowly conducting isthmus between the tricuspid valve ring and the inferior vena cava (Figure 5.8). Once conduction is no longer possible over this isthmus, the stable re-entrant circuit can no longer form. Using current ablation techniques, success rate for this procedure is equal to that of catheter ablation of accessory pathways and AV nodal tachycardia.

Further reading

Bauernfeind RA, Amat-y-Leon F, Chingra RC, et al. Chronic nonparoxysmal sinus tachycardia in otherwise healthy persons. Ann Intern Med 1979;91:702–710.

Cosio FG, Arribas F, Palacios J, et al. Fragmented electrograms and continuous electrical activity in atrial flutter. Am J Cardiol 1986;57:1309–1314.

Haines DE, DiMarco JP. Sustained intra-atrial re-entrant tachycardia: clinical, electrocardiographic and electrophysiologic characteristics and long-term follow-up. J Am Coll Cardiol 1990;15:1345–1354.

Saoudi N, Atallah G, Cheng P-S, et al. Radiofrequency catheter ablation for the treatment of human type I atrial flutter. Identification of a critical zone in the re-entrant circuit by endocardial mapping techniques. Circulation 1992;86:1233–1240.

Shah DC, Haissaguerre M, Jais P, et al. Atrial flutter; contemporary electrophysiology and catheter ablation. PACE 1999;22:344–359.

Wu D, Amat-y-Leon F, Denes P, et al. Demonstration of sustained sinus and atrial re-entry as a mechanism of paroxysmal supraventricular tachycardia. Circulation 1975;51:234–243.

6: Atrial fibrillation

Atrial fibrillation (AF) is the most common cardiac arrhythmia worldwide, with a prevalence of approximately 1% in the overall population, rising to 4% in the over-65s. It is associated with considerable mortality and morbidity, principally due to the consequences of stroke and heart failure. It currently represents the greatest challenge to the cardiological community of any of the cardiac arrhythmias in terms of understanding its mechanism and devising appropriate therapy.

Patterns of clinical presentation

Most patients who first develop atrial fibrillation have symptoms of irregular palpitations, the severity of which is dependent upon the ventricular rate during tachycardia. Syncope is very rare but shortness of breath not infrequent. Patients with atrial fibrillation and a well-controlled or slow ventricular rate may be asymptomatic or present with a complication such as stroke.

- *Single episode*: Atrial fibrillation may be due to a precipitating cause (cardiac surgery, chest infection, pulmonary embolus, electrolyte disturbance), and once this cause has been eliminated AF does not return.
- *Paroxysmal atrial fibrillation*: In this form of atrial fibrillation the episodes of arrhythmia are self-terminating and recurrent . This starts typically in the 50s or 60s age group but can occur earlier. If paroxysms of atrial fibrillation are going to self-terminate they usually do so within 24–48 hours. This condition is associated with mitral valve disease, ischaemic heart disease and thyrotoxicosis as well as a number of rarer conditions (Table 6.1). In addition, many patients have no underlying detectable cause or structural heart disease; this is termed idiopathic or "lone" atrial fibrillation.
- *Persistent atrial fibrillation*: Describes episodes of arrhythmia that are not self-terminating and require drugs or DC cardioversion for their termination.
- *Permanent atrial fibrillation*: Describes the situation in which the patient is in continuous atrial fibrillation that cannot be terminated at all.

The terms *chronic* or *established* atrial fibrillation are frequently used in the literature and refer to long-standing atrial fibrillation that has not self-terminated, i.e. covers the persistent and permanent forms.

Table 6.1   Causes of atrial fibrillation.

Conditions causing demonstrable structural change to the atria

1. Raised atrial pressure
   - Mitral or tricuspid valve disease – rheumatic and other
   - Ventricular disease causing systolic or diastolic dysfunction
     - coronary artery disease
     - aortic/pulmonary valve disease
     - cardiomyopathy
   - Systemic or pulmonary hypertension (inc. pulmonary embolism)
2. Atrial ischaemia
   - Coronary artery disease
3. Atrial inflammation/infiltration
   - Pericarditis, postcardiotomy syndrome
   - Amyloidosis, sarcoidosis, haemochromatosis
   - Myocarditis
   - Primary tumour, direct spread or metastasis of other tumour
4. Age-related changes
   - Atrial fibrosis
5. Other
   - Congenital heart disease, especially atrial septal defect
   - Cardiac trauma

Conditions not causing demonstrable structural change to the atria

1. Sympathetic stimulation
   - Hyperthyroidism
   - Pheochromocytoma
   - Anxiety
   - Ethanol, caffeine, stimulant drugs
   - "Adrenergic" paroxysmal atrial fibrillation
2. Parasympathetic stimulation
   - "Vagal" paroxysmal atrial fibrillation
3. Toxic effects
   - Ethanol, carbon monoxide, drugs, chemicals
4. Neurological
   - Subarachnoid haemorrhage
5. Other
   - Hypoxia, pneumonia
   - Idiopathic atrial fibrillation

(*From* Murgatroyd FD and Camm AJ *Atrial fibrillation for the clinician.* Armonk, NY: Futura, 1995.)

Mechanisms

Atrial fibrillation was described soon after the invention of the electrocardiogram in the late 1800s. Although a number of possible mechanisms were discussed, it became generally accepted that the arrhythmia was due to chaotic and random atrial activation in which the whole of the atrium was activated incoordinately. In 1985 Allessie *et al* demonstrated that, contrary to this contention, during atrial fibrillation the atria appear to be activated by several separate "wavelets" of activity which meander around the atrium re-exciting areas that had previously been electrically silent (Figure 6.1). This experimental work was confirmation of a hypothesis put forward by Moe postulating that stability of atrial fibrillation was related to the number of such wavelets that could be accommodated by the atrial tissue. A consequence of this hypothesis is that stability of atrial fibrillation is related to the size of these wavelets relative to the size of the atria. The size of the wavelets is influenced by the electrophysiological properties of the atrium, a smaller wavelet size occurring in the presence of shorter atrial refractoriness, and slower atrial conduction. These wavelets represent a form of functional re-entry, usually considered to be via a leading circle or more likely a spiral wave mechanism (see Chapter 3).

More recently (1997), Haissaguerre has described a form of atrial fibrillation in patients in which there is a discrete "origin" of the arrhythmia, nearly always sited at the junction of the pulmonary veins and left atrial musculature. Although the exact mechanism is unknown, there are some characteristics suggestive of triggered activity. There is experimental evidence to indicate that rapid atrial activation by such an atrial source may lead to a decrease in atrial refractoriness throughout the atrium (atrial electrical remodelling) and this may lead to a self-perpetuation of arrhythmia ("AF begets AF") and maintenance due to the development of multiple small wavelets. The increased prevalence of AF in the elderly is likely to be due at least in part to the frequency of underlying pathologies. In addition, age-related changes in the atria include an increase in fibrous and adipose tissue. It is likely that the development of fibrous tissue between atrial cells increases the likelihood of slow and inhomogenous conduction, thereby facilitating the generation of functional re-entrant circuits and AF.

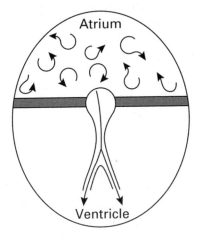

Figure 6.1   Schematic diagram of re-entrant "wavelets" underlying atrial fibrillation.

There is a familial form of atrial fibrillation which is now becoming increasingly recognised. Although a number of loci for the relevant genes have been identified, the precise nature of the genetic abnormality is uncertain as yet.

Electrocardiographic features and diagnosis

- Atrial fibrillation typically presents as a narrow complex irregular tachycardia in which no P waves are evident between the QRS complexes. Usually, irregular low amplitude f waves are evident (Figure 6.2).
- Ventricular complexes may be broad in the presence of bundle branch block (Figure 6.3) or conduction down an accessory pathway (see Chapter 15). In the latter situation ventricular rate may be very rapid and the patient severely haemodynamically compromised (Figure 6.4).
- Patients with the relatively rare "focal" form of AF may show frequent bursts of AF in which the f waves appear to be more organised and sometimes have the appearance of atrial flutter (Figure 6.5).

Complications of AF

AF associated with significant mitral valve disease in the absence of anticoagulation is associated with an 18-fold increase in the risk of systemic embolism, principally stroke. Non-valvular AF with other risk factors (structural heart disease, hypertension, age >65, diabetes) increases the risk by approximately five times above normal. Young patients with no structural heart disease or other risk factor have a negligible increase in risk for embolic events, if any.

Other complications of AF

A sustained rapid ventricular rate can, over periods of time (weeks and months), give rise to left ventricular dysfunction. As with other causes of "tachycardia-related cardiomyopathy", this dysfunction is usually reversible once the arrhythmia is terminated or the ventricular rate is brought under control. Left ventricular failure or syncope are unusual with acute episodes of AF, although certainly can occur in the presence of structural abnormalities of the ventricles such as hypertrophic or ischaemic cardiomyopathy.

Prognosis

Atrial fibrillation has frequently in the past been considered as a benign condition. However, it is estimated that the presence of this arrhythmia is associated with a doubling of mortality over similar patients without atrial fibrillation. The prognosis depends primarily on the underlying cause of the arrhythmia and the degree of coexistent structural heart disease. Patients with structurally normal hearts (idiopathic or lone AF) have an excellent prognosis that is little different from normal. It should be noted that although atrial fibrillation in the setting of structural heart disease is associated with

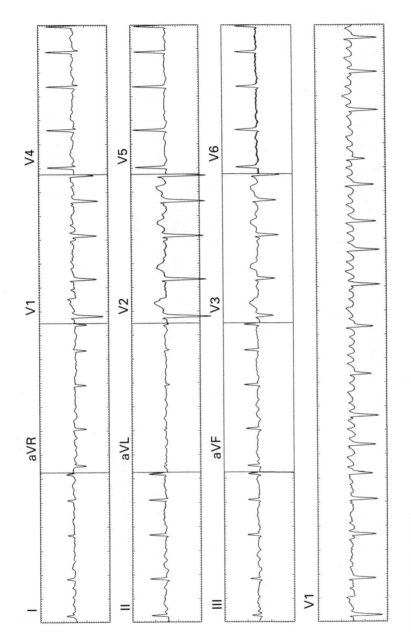
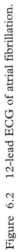

Figure 6.2   12-lead ECG of atrial fibrillation.

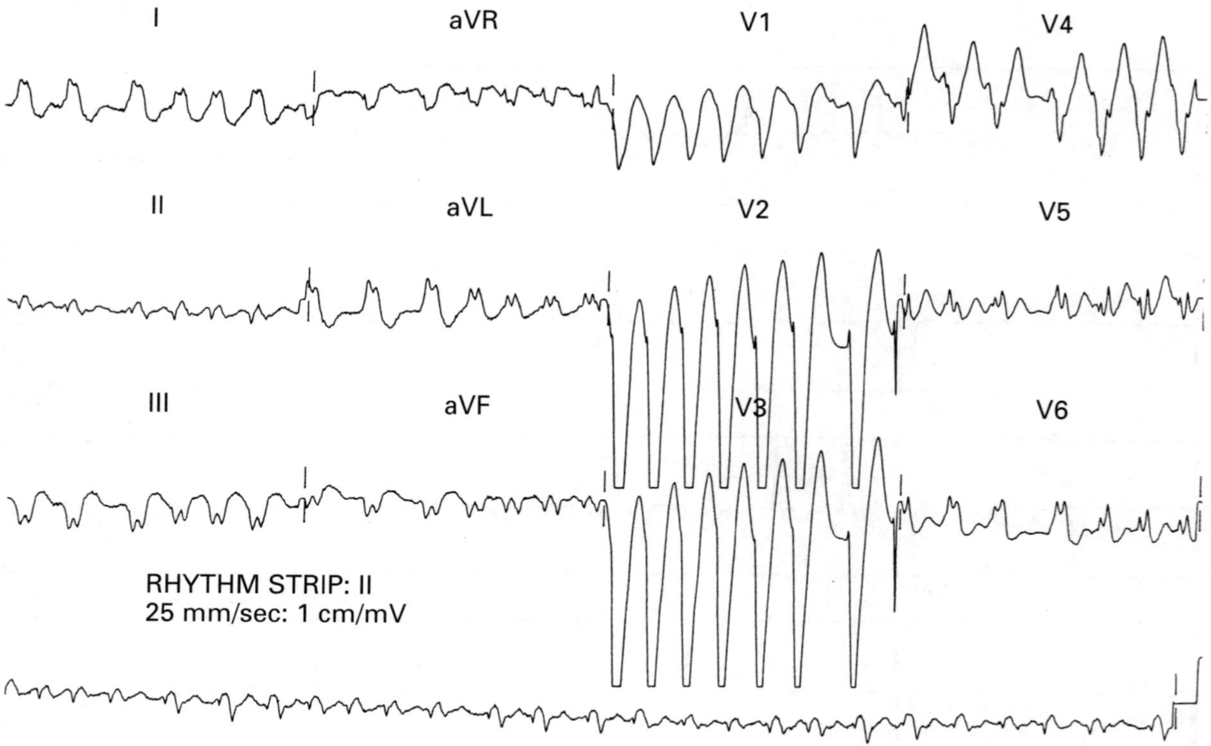

Figure 6.3   12-lead ECG of AF in the setting of pre-existing bundle branch block.

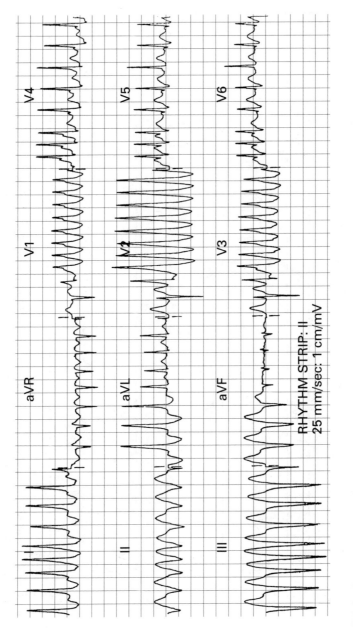

RHYTHM STRIP: II
25 mm/sec; 1 cm/mV

Figure 6.4   12-lead ECG of "pre-excited AF": AF with conduction to the ventricles via an accessory pathway.

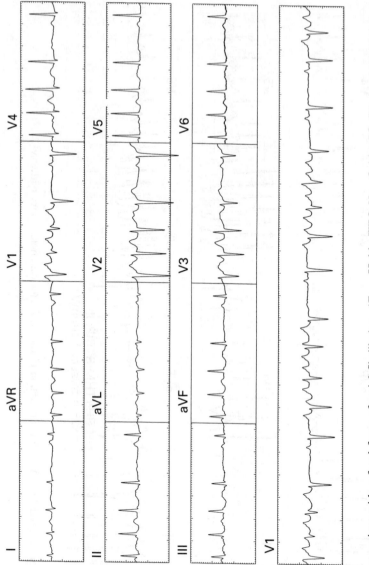

Figure 6.5 "Bursts" of AF in a patient with a focal form of atrial fibrillation. (*From* Hobbs WJC, Van Gelder IC, Fitzpatrick AP, Crijns HJGM, Garratt CJ. The role of atrial electrical remodeling in the progression of focal atrial ectopy to persistent atrial fibrillation. *J Cardiovasc Electrophysiol* 1999;**10**:866–70.)

increased mortality, there is no hard evidence as yet that this increase in mortality is negated by subsequent return and maintenance of sinus rhythm.

Anticoagulation therapy

Evidence from several large randomised placebo controlled trials has demonstrated that warfarin prevents stroke and improves survival in patients with atrial fibrillation in high risk groups, i.e. over 65, in the presence of structural heart disease, hypertension, or diabetes. Most of the patients in these trials had long-standing atrial fibrillation but patients with paroxysmal atrial fibrillation were also included. INR should be maintained between 2 and 3. Young patients with normal echocardiograms are at very low risk of embolic events and in these patients the risk of embolic stroke is outweighed by the risk of warfarin therapy. Aspirin is frequently prescribed for this group, although it is uncertain that this confers any benefit.

Patients undergoing cardioversion of AF of more than 48 hours' duration are at risk of dislodgement of atrial thrombus and embolic stroke. Two alternative strategies may be followed to avoid this complication (Figure 6.6). It is usually recommended that patients are anticoagulated with warfarin (INR between 2 and 3) for three weeks prior to any attempt at cardioversion and for four weeks following cardioversion, as it is known that cardioversion is associated with an increased risk of embolic events. The rationale for the relatively long pretreatment with warfarin is (a) prevention of the *development* of atrial thrombus and (b) to allow time for any thrombi that are present to resolve or become organised. An alternative strategy is to perform a

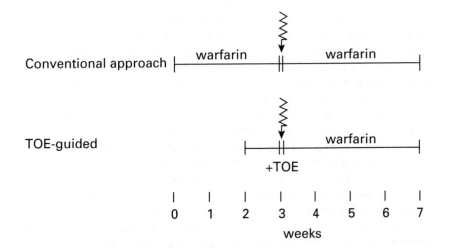

Figure 6.6 Conventional and transoesophageal-guided approaches to DC cardioversion of AF. The pre-cardioversion warfarinisation period can be reduced or eliminated by the use of TOE, but post-cardioversion warfarin is still required.

51

transoesophageal echocardiogram (TOE) immediately prior to cardioversion to exclude any left atrial or left atrial appendage thrombus. If this alternative strategy is used, the patient should be heparinised at the time of cardioversion. The rationale for the continuation of anticoagulation after cardioversion is that there is good evidence that the thrombogenic tendency persists for approximately four weeks after return of sinus rhythm. Anticoagulation should be given in the post-cardioversion period even if transoesophageal echocardiography has excluded a thrombus; there is evidence that thrombi may develop in the immediate post-cardioversion period when atrial contraction remains impaired.

Therapy directed to the arrhythmia itself

Antiarrhythmic strategies aimed at atrial fibrillation can be considered in two groups: those that attempt to maintain the patient in sinus rhythm and those that attempt to control ventricular rate. In general, it is considered that maintenance of sinus rhythm, if possible, is preferable although clear data in terms of mortality benefit are lacking at present. Long term strategies are discussed below, and therapy of the acute arrhythmia is discussed in Chapter 15.

Attempts to maintain sinus rhythm

Antiarrhythmic drugs

In patients with paroxysmal atrial fibrillation, treatment with antiarrhythmic drugs is often on a "trial and error" basis, with different drugs being tried in an attempt to reduce the frequency of attacks. Beta blockade is often tried in the first instance, particularly if there is any evidence of relationship between attacks and exercise. If the paroxysms appear to be vagally mediated (occur when relaxed, or after a long pause seen on a 24 hour tape), then disopyramide is thought to be of some benefit. The best evidence of benefit is that for patients treated with flecainide or propafenone, both of which have been shown to increase time to recurrence of paroxysmal AF in placebo controlled trials (Figure 6.7). These drugs should not be prescribed to patients with impaired ventricular function or ischaemic heart disease however (see Chapter 16). Quinidine was once a favourite drug for the treatment of atrial fibrillation in the UK (and still is relatively widely used in the USA), but evidence drawn from a number of studies has indicated that the drug may increase mortality in the general AF population. It is thought that this effect may relate to a proarrhythmic effect in the setting of structural heart disease that is common to agents of Vaughan Williams class 1 (see Chapter 16). In the setting of structural heart disease, amiodarone is probably the most effective drug, with a maintenance dose of 200 mg a day minimising the likelihood of long term adverse effects. Digoxin is commonly used in patients with paroxysmal AF despite evidence that it does not reduce the frequency of paroxysms to any clinically

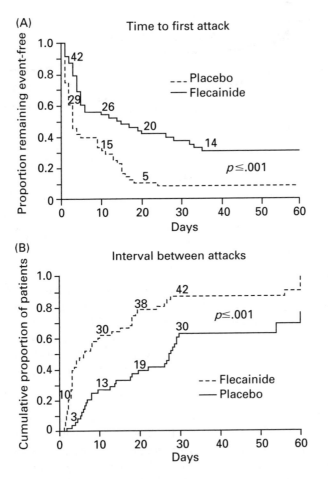

Figure 6.7   The beneficial effect of flecainide on time to first attack (*A*) and interval between attacks of paroxysmal AF (*B*) in a randomised placebo controlled trial. (*From* Andersen JL, Gilbert EM, Alpert BL *et al*. Prevention of symptomatic recurrences of paroxysmal atrial fibrillation in patients initially tolerating antiarrhythmic therapy. *Circulation* 1989;**80**:1557–70.)

significant extent. The drug does lower ventricular rate during the paroxysms, however.

Patients with persistent atrial fibrillation have a very high likelihood of relapsing within the first week or two following cardioversion (see below), and one year following cardioversion about 50% of patients remain in sinus rhythm. There is evidence that this number can be increased to a degree by the use of beta blockade after cardioversion and to a greater degree by long term therapy with amiodarone (Figure 6.8).

Atrial fibrillation occurs in up to 30% of patients following cardiac surgery and not infrequently prolongs hospital stay in these patients. There are many potential causes of the arrhythmia in such patients, including the

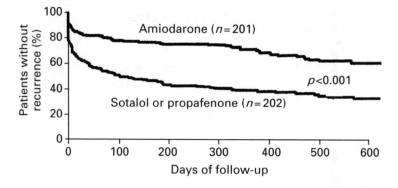

Figure 6.8 Beneficial effect of amiodarone versus other drugs in maintaining sinus rhythm following cardioversion of AF. (*From* the CTAF trial, Roy D, Talajic M, Dorian P *et al*. Amiodarone to prevent recurrence of atrial fibrillation. *N Engl J Med* 2000; **342**:913–20.)

direct effect of trauma and pericardial reaction. The behaviour of this form of AF does appear different from other forms however. In particular it is thought to be "adrenergically-driven", the incidence following the post-operative rise in circulating catecholamines and peaking at two to three days postoperatively. Peri- and postoperative beta blockade with propranolol, acebutolol or timolol is associated with a lower incidence of AF postoperatively.

DC cardioversion

Electrical methods to terminate AF were first described in the early 1960s and are the most effective means of restoring sinus rhythm in patients with persistent AF. External DC cardioversion is the most common method: the technique involves the delivery of a high energy depolarising shock between two electrode paddles placed on the external surface of the chest. Synchronous depolarisation of all atrial cells is followed (if successful) by synchronous repolarisation and resumption of normal sinus rhythm. The usual convention is to place one paddle over the base of the heart (at the level of the upper sternum or right parasternal area) and the other over the apex. The alternative configuration is known as anteroposterior (one electrode placed anteriorly over the sternum, one placed posteriorly over the spine). The most important technical factor for success is good skin contact with adequately gelled electrodes with the avoidance of "short-circuiting" due to excess gel between the paddles. Reliable synchronisation of the cardioverison shock with the R wave is essential for safe cardioversion, since ventricular fibrillation can easily be provoked by a shock falling in the vulnerable period of ventricular repolarisation. Some published protocols suggest starting with low energy shocks, increasing in energy if these fail. Energies of less than 200 J are rarely effective for the cardioversion of AF, however, and it is sensible to start with energies of at least this amount. Relative contraindications to DC cardioversion are digoxin toxicity (not just the fact that the patient is taking digoxin), particularly in the presence of hypokalaemia, as the risk of ventricular arrhythmias is significantly increased. Success rates vary between 70% and 95% and are related primarily to the preceding duration of AF: the less time the patient has been in AF the more likely is successful return to sinus rhythm.

There is evidence that success of cardioversion (both in terms of initial return to sinus rhythm and subsequent maintenance of sinus rhythm) is increased if the patient has been loaded with amiodarone prior to the cardioversion and certainly this may be attempted if "drug-free" cardioversion has been unsuccessful. External cardioversion has limited efficacy in patients with very large chests and in these patients the alternative technique of internal cardioversion is particularly useful. In this technique the DC shock is delivered between electrode catheters inserted into the right atrium and coronary sinus (or alternatively left pulmonary artery) (Figure 6.9). Much less energy is required for successful cardioversion as none is dissipated in the chest wall and musculature. As with external cardioversion, however, the technique is limited by the relatively high incidence of AF recurrence following the procedure. Nevertheless, the strategy of occasional repeated cardioversion (internal or external) of patients with recurrent episodes of persistent AF can be a useful adjunct to antiarrhythmic therapy. An extrapolation of this strategy forms the basis for the use of the implantable atrial defibrillator. This form of therapy is useful for the occasional patient with episodes of persistent AF that are not too frequent, do not self-terminate and are associated with haemodynamic compromise.

Catheter ablation procedures

Catheter ablation techniques can be curative for patients with focal forms of atrial fibrillation. These patients usually have a "source" of their atrial fibrillation at the junction of the pulmonary veins with the left atrial musculature. For this approach to be successful currently one needs to be able to "map" the origin of the fibrillation, using either the onset of bursts of AF or using atrial premature beats as markers of the source (Figure 6.10). Newer techniques are being developed so that such sites can be targeted "blind", i.e. without the need for the presence of spontaneous AF or premature beats at the time of the procedure. A different ablation approach to the cure of AF is the use of long linear lesions to divide the atrial mass sufficiently to limit wavelet propagation. To date this approach has not been very successful.

Maze procedure

This is the surgical equivalent of (and preceded) the long linear ablation approach in which the atria are dissected and sutured in an attempt to limit the size of electrically continuous atria (Figure 6.11). It is significantly more successful than the catheter ablation method in terms of maintenance of sinus rhythm but, as it requires thoracotomy, it is associated with some morbidity. In general it is reserved at present for patients undergoing surgery for other reasons, for example mitral valve replacement.

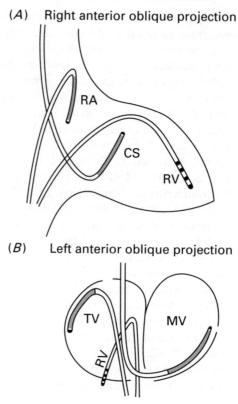

(A)   Right anterior oblique projection

(B)   Left anterior oblique projection

Figure 6.9   Catheter positions for internal cardioversion of AF. The right and left oblique radiographic projections are those most commonly used in the positioning of these catheters. A low energy shock is delivered between the right atrial and coronary sinus electrodes, maximising the amount of atrial tissue subjected to a depolarising shock. (CS = coronary sinus, MV = mitral valve ring, TV = tricuspid valve ring, RA = right atrial catheter, RV = right ventricular catheter)

Pacemaker therapy

There are theoretical reasons to believe that consistently increasing the atrial rate in patients with paroxysmal AF might reduce the susceptibility to AF by reducing inhomogeneities of repolarisation and perhaps suppressing the generation of atrial ectopic beats. Indeed, some trials of permanent atrial-based pacing in this population have demonstrated statistically significant benefit. The reduction in frequency of episodes is not marked however, and this form of therapy is, in general, only recommended in patients with a documented and consistent bradycardia-dependent form of AF, i.e. ambulatory monitoring demonstrates that AF initiation is preceded by bradycardia. A number of cardiologists follow a policy of implanting a pacemaker some time prior to an AV nodal ablation procedure (see below) and cancel the ablation procedure itself if the patient shows significant improvement with pacemaker treatment alone. My own

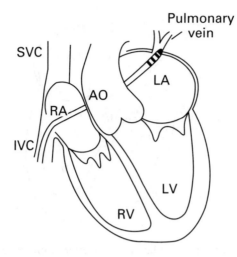

Figure 6.10   Schematic representation of ablation catheter position for cure of focal AF. Transeptal puncture is required for access to the left atrium.

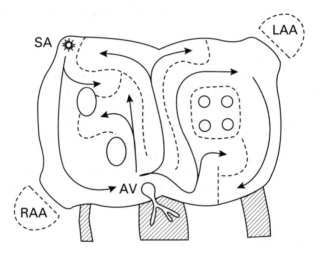

Figure 6.11   Schematic representations of the incisions (dotted lines) and route of atrial activation (solid arrows) in the Maze operation. (*From* Murgatroyd F, Camm AJ. *Atrial fibrillation for the clinician*. Armonk, NY: Futura, 1995.)

experience is that this policy is rarely successful in the medium to long term.

Control of ventricular rate

Antiarrhythmic drugs
The most widely used agents for the long term control of ventricular rate during atrial fibrillation are digoxin and/or verapamil. In many patients

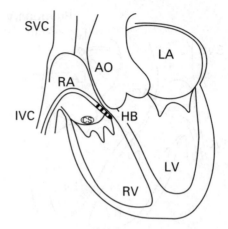

Figure 6.12   Schematic representation of ablation catheter position in a His bundle ablation procedure.

these agents are useful in controlling the ventricular rate (to less than 100 beats/min) at rest but beta blockers are often necessary to blunt the abnormally high rate response to exercise.

AV node ablation and pacing

If medical therapy is unsuccessful in terms of controlling the ventricular rate, ablation of the AV node/His bundle (Figure 6.12) is a very successful technique in terms of suppressing symptoms of palpitations and reversing any rate-related deterioration of ventricular function. Following His bundle ablation a ventricular escape rhythm is present in most patients but must be considered unreliable and the patient potentially pacemaker-dependent. Those with significant periods of sinus rhythm require dual chamber pacing with mode switching capability. Those who are in atrial fibrillation all the time should receive ventricular pacemakers with rate response (VVIR).

Further reading

Allessie MA, Lammers WJEP, Bonke FIM. Experimental evaluation of Moe's multiple wavelet hypothesis of atrial fibrillation. In: Zipes DP, Jalife J (eds). *Cardiac electrophysiology and arrhythmias.* Orlando, FL: Grune & Stratton, 1985, 265–75.

Brugada R, Tapscott T, Czernuszewicz, *et al.* Identification of a genetic locus for familial atrial fibrillation. *N Engl J Med* 1997;**336**(13):905–11.

Jais P, Haissaugerre M, Shah D, *et al.* A focal source of atrial fibrillation treated by discrete radiofrequency ablation. *Circulation* 1997;**95**:572–6.

Scheinman MM, Morady F, Hess DS, *et al.* Catheter-induced ablation of the atrioventricular function to control refractory supraventricular arrhythmia. *JAMA* 1982;**248**:851.

Wijffels MCEF, Kirchof CJHJ, Dorland R, Allessie MA. Atrial fibrillation begets atrial fibrillation: a study in awake chronically instrumented goats. *Circulation* 1995;**92**:1954–68.

7: Junctional tachycardias

Definition

Junctional tachycardias are those in which the tachycardia circuit involves the AV junction. The two principal forms of junctional tachycardia are AV nodal re-entrant tachycardia and AV re-entrant tachycardia using an accessory AV connection. In both of these situations a re-entrant tachycardia circuit exists which is anatomically fixed.

Mechanism

Atrioventricular nodal re-entrant tachycardia (AVNRT) is a form of congenital re-entrant tachycardia in which the re-entrant circuit involves the AV node and perinodal atrium. In the common type of AVNRT, conduction occurs down a slow AV nodal pathway in an antegrade (atrium to ventricle) direction and returns via a fast AV nodal pathway in a retrograde (ventricle to atrium) direction (Figure 7.1). The fast pathway is thought to be sited anatomically cranial to the compact AV node and the slow pathway more posteriorly towards the opening of the coronary sinus into the right

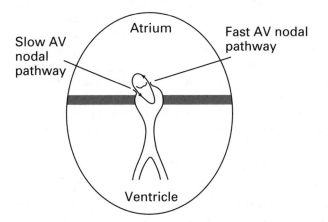

Figure 7.1   In the common type of AVNRT, conduction occurs down a slow AV nodal pathway in an antegrade (atrium to ventricle) direction and returns via a fast AV nodal pathway in a retrograde (ventricle to atrium) direction. (*From* Garratt CJ, Griffith MJ. *Electrocardiographic diagnosis of tachycardias.* Armonk, NY: Futura, 1994.)

59

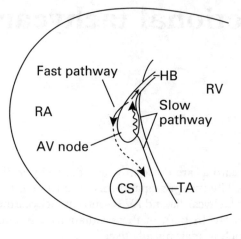

Figure 7.2   Postulated anatomical positions of the fast and slow AV nodal pathways. The structures are orientated as seen from a PA radiographic projection, as with a standard chest *x* ray. CS = coronary sinus, HB = his bundle, TA = tricuspid annulus. (*From* Jackman WM *et al*. Treatment of supraventricular tachycardia due to atrioventricular nodal reentry by radiofrequency catheter ablation of slow-pathway conduction. *NEJM* 1992;**327**:313–8.)

atrium (Figure 7.2). In the atypical form of AVNRT (about 10% of cases), the re-entrant circuit travels in the reverse direction, i.e. antegradely down the fast pathway, retrogradely up the slow pathway.

   Atrioventricular re-entrant tachycardia involves an anatomically fixed re-entrant circuit utilising the AV node and accessory AV connection or pathway, and the intervening areas of atrial and ventricular myocardium. In the common orthodromic form, antegrade conduction occurs via the AV node and retrograde conduction via the accessory pathway (Figure 7.3). In the rare antidromic form (approximately 10%) the circuit travels in the reverse direction. The site of the accessory pathway, which is only a millimetre or so in width and 4 or 5 mm in length, can be almost anywhere on the AV ring but is most commonly on the lateral side of the left AV ring. In approximately 10% of cases more than one accessory pathway is present. In this situation it is possible that the re-entrant circuit may involve both pathways without the AV node being involved at all (Figure 7.4).

Patterns of clinical presentation

Wolff–Parkinson–White syndrome

Patients with junctional tachycardia may first seek medical attention once the tachycardia has subsided. If an accessory pathway is present, its presence may be inferred from the existence of a delta wave on the surface electrocardiogram, which represents pre-excitation of the ventricles, i.e. early and abnormal activation of the ventricle via the pathway during sinus rhythm (Figure 7.5). Patients are usually in their teens or 20s at presentation.

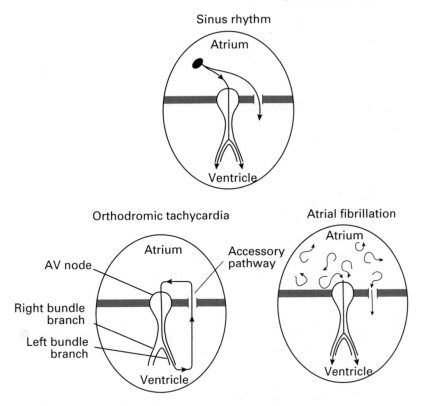

Figure 7.3   Patterns of ventricular and atrial activation in the Wolff–Parkinson–White syndrome. During sinus rhythm the ventricle is activated (pre-excited) via an accessory pathway as well as via the AV node, leading to the appearance of the characteristic delta wave on the surface ECG. During orthodromic tachycardia antegrade conduction occurs via the AV node/His–Purkinje system (resulting in a narrow QRS complex) and retrograde conduction occurs via the accessory pathway. During atrial fibrillation conduction to the ventricles occurs via both the AV node and the accessory pathway, leading to both narrow and wide complexes and fusion beats (a combination of the two).

Narrow complex regular tachycardia (Figures 7.6 and 7.7)

In general, these forms of tachycardia are well tolerated by the patient, not least because in the main they occur in young patients with normal ventricles. Syncope, if it occurs, usually does so at the onset of tachycardia when blood pressure is low and before reflex vasoconstriction has returned blood pressure to near normal levels (see Figure 14.1).

Patients with accessory pathways may develop atrial fibrillation

If the accessory pathway conducts in an antegrade direction, this may be conducted to the ventricles at a very rapid rate (Figure 7.8). This is a dangerous situation and ventricular fibrillation and death may occur if the

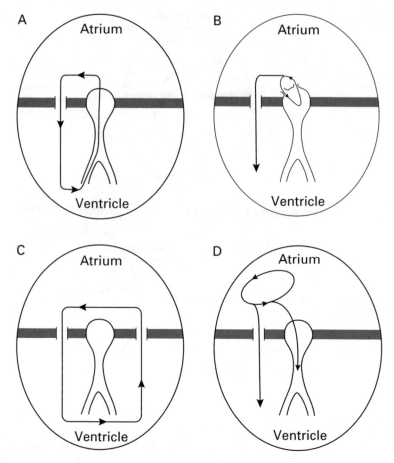

Figure 7.4 A variety of re-entrant arrhythmias associated with the WPW syndrome and producing wide complex regular tachycardia. In each case the ventricle is activated via an accessory pathway, producing a wide (pre-excited) QRS complex. (*A*) Antidromic tachycardia; (*B*) AVNRT with "bystander" activation of an accessory pathway; (*C*) tachycardia involving two accessory pathways and excluding the AV node; (*D*) atrial flutter with activation of the ventricle via an accessory pathway. (*From* Garratt CJ, Griffith MJ. *Electrocardiographic diagnosis of tachycardias*. Armonk, NY: Futura, 1994.)

ventricular rates are sufficiently high. It should be noted that not all patients with accessory pathways have antegrade conduction to the ventricles and a delta wave during sinus rhythm. In many patients conduction only occurs via the accessory pathway in a retrograde direction and in this situation the pathways are said to be "concealed".

Tachycardia mediated cardiomyopathy

Occasionally junctional tachycardias may be persistent or incessant rather than paroxysmal (Figure 7.9), and in this situation (tachycardia continuing

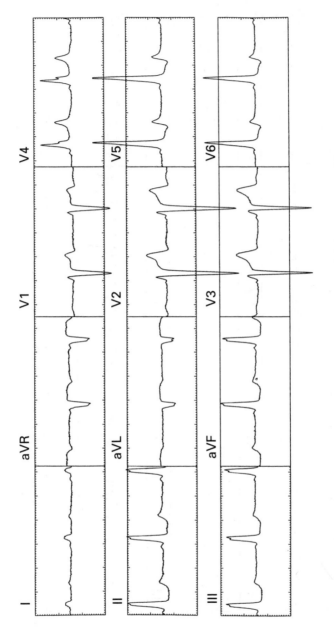

Figure 7.5   Surface ECG in a patient with the WPW syndrome. The short PR interval and delta wave are evident.

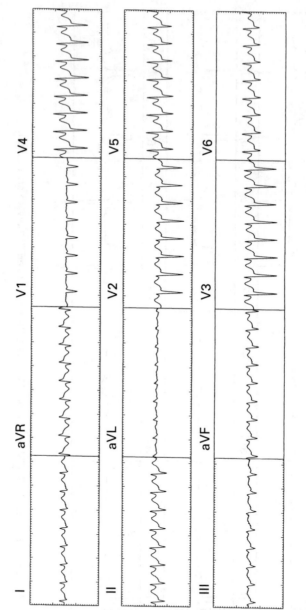

Figure 7.6   12-lead ECG during AVNRT. No clear retrograde P waves can be identified, but the pseudo RSR pattern in lead V1 is suggestive of retrograde atrial activation occurring almost immediately after ventricular activation.

Figure 7.7 12-lead ECG of orthodromic tachycardia. Retrograde atrial activation can be identified as a "retrograde P wave" shortly after the QRS complex. Alternation of QRS amplitude can be seen particularly in leads V3–V5 and is most commonly seen (but not exclusively) in orthodromic tachycardia.

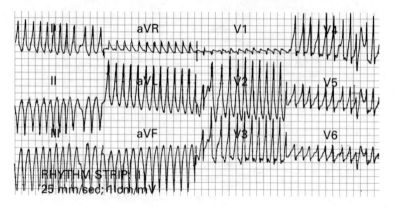

Figure 7.8 12-lead ECG of pre-excited atrial fibrillation in a patient with the WPW syndrome.

for days, weeks, and perhaps months) there may be a progressive impairment of ventricular function. If the tachycardia rate is relatively slow, then the patient may not complain of palpitations but may present in heart failure. This is a very important cause of heart failure to recognise in that it is potentially completely curable.

Diagnosis

Surface electrocardiogram

Diagnosis can be made to a large extent from the surface electrocardiogram (Chapter 15). The site as well as the presence of an accessory pathway can be inferred from the presence and pattern of pre-excitation on the electrocardiogram. Patients with the common left-sided accessory pathways have a dominant R wave in leads V1 and V2. The position of the pathway is relevant in so far as it is of some help in planning the appropriate ablation procedure (see Chapter 17).

Electrophysiology study

The principal means of diagnosis of junctional tachycardia at electrophysiology study is the use of electrode catheters to determine the earliest site of atrial activation during tachycardia induced by ventricular or atrial extrastimuli. Earliest atrial activation close to the bundle of His strongly suggests AV nodal tachycardia (particularly if atrial and ventricular activation is nearly synchronous) whereas earliest atrial activation at a site distant to the AV node indicates the presence of an accessory pathway (see Chapter 17).

Prognosis

- Patients with AV nodal tachycardia or AV re-entrant tachycardia using a concealed accessory pathway are thought to have a normal prognosis.

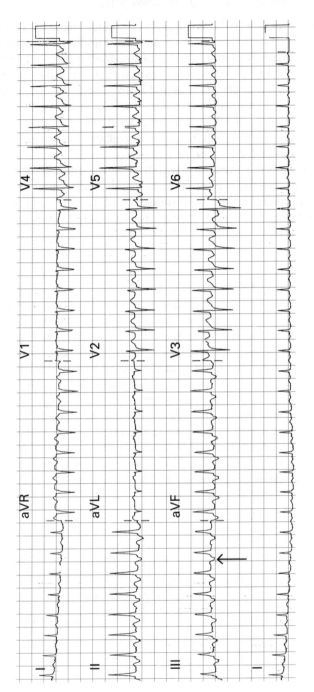

Figure 7.9 Incessant orthodromic tachycardia associated with retrograde atrial activation, via a slowly conducting accessory pathway with a "long RP" interval (*arrowed*) during tachycardia. Tachycardias such as this are sometimes referred to as "permanent junctional re-entrant tachycardia" or PJRT.

- Patients with accessory pathways capable of conducting in an antegrade direction are potentially at risk of death from rapidly conducted atrial fibrillation, although even in this group deaths from WPW syndrome are rare. Electrophysiologic studies in patients with WPW syndrome reveal that all those that have been resuscitated from sudden death are capable of conducting atrial fibrillation at a rate of 280 beats/min (shortest RR intervals less than 250 msec), at least for a short period of time. Patients who are not capable of conducting atrial fibrillation at such a rate are considered to have a "safe" accessory pathway.
- Patients with the WPW syndrome who have never suffered palpitations are, as a group, very unlikely to conduct atrial fibrillation at very rapid rates. As a consequence, the risk of sudden death is very very low in this group and investigation and treatment is not advised unless there are special occupational reasons.

Therapy

Radiofrequency catheter ablation

Radiofrequency catheter ablation is first line treatment for patients with symptoms of palpitations in the Wolff–Parkinson–White syndrome. Electrode catheters are inserted into the heart via the inferior vena cava or retrogradely via the ascending aorta and radiofrequency energy applied to the tip of the electrode catheter either at the site of earliest atrial activation during tachycardia or earliest ventricular activation during sinus rhythm (Figure 7.10). The procedure has a success rate approaching 95% and is performed under local anaesthetic. Risks (less than 1%) include embolic events (for left-sided pathways), AV block (for septal pathways), and tamponade.

In patients with AVNRT a more anatomically guided approach to catheter ablation is usually undertaken. The electrode catheter is positioned with its tip at the site of the anatomical slow pathway and radiofrequency

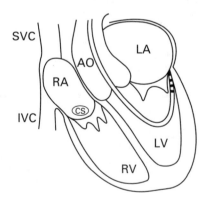

Figure 7.10   Schematic diagram of a typical (subvalvar) position of an ablation catheter using the retrograde transaortic approach for ablation of left-sided accessory pathways.

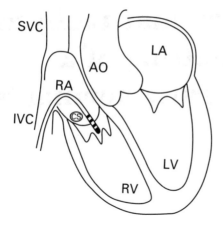

Figure 7.11 Typical "anatomical" catheter position for ablation of the AV nodal slow pathway.

energy delivered at this site (Figure 7.11). As with accessory pathways, the rate of procedural success is very high but the risk of AV block is somewhat higher (approximately 2%) due to the proximity of the compact AV node to the ablation site.

Antiarrhythmic drug therapy

Patients with AVNRT or orthodromic AV re-entrant tachycardia using a concealed accessory pathway may choose to have a trial of antiarrhythmic drug therapy prior to or instead of a catheter ablation procedure. Verapamil or beta blockade is usually prescribed in the first instance, although flecainide is likely to be more effective.

Further reading

Jackman WM, Beckman KJ, McClelland JH, *et al*. Treatment of supraventricular tachycardia due to atrioventricular nodal reentry by radiofrequency catheter ablation of slow pathway conduction. *N Engl J Med* 1992;**327**:313–18.

Jackman WM, Xunzhang W, Friday KH, *et al*. Catheter ablation of accessory atrioventricular pathways (Wolff–Parkinson–White syndrome) by radiofrequency current. *N Engl J Med* 1991;**324**:1605–11.

Klein GJ, Bashore TM, Sellers TD, *et al*. Ventricular fibrillation in the Wolff–Parkinson–White syndrome. *Circulation* 1974;**49**:22.

Leitch JW, Klein GJ, Yee R. Prognostic value of electrophysiology testing in asymptomatic patients with Wolff–Parkinson–White syndrome. *Circulation* 1990;**82**:1718.

Prystowsky EN. Diagnosis and management of the pre-excitation syndrome. *Curr Probl Cardiol* 1988;**12**:230.

Wolff L, Parkinson J, White P, *et al*. Bundle branch block with short P–R interval in healthy young people prone to paroxysmal tachycardia. *Am Heart J* 1930;**5**:685.

8: Ventricular tachycardia in the setting of a structurally normal heart

In about 10% of cases of sustained ventricular tachycardia (VT) left ventricular function is normal and there is no associated coronary disease or any form of cardiomyopathy. At least two distinct forms can be identified (see below). Although these forms of tachycardia are often referred to as "idiopathic", we do know a great deal about their underlying mechanisms.

Right ventricular outflow tract VT ("adenosine-sensitive VT") (RVOT)

Approximately 80% of cases of "idiopathic" VT originate in the outflow tract of the right ventricle.

Clinical presentation, surface ECG, and diagnostic tests

Forms of clinical presentation range from frequent bursts of monomorphic ventricular extrasystoles to paroxysms of sustained VT. This arrhythmia may be precipitated or exacerbated by exercise. The presenting symptom is nearly always palpitation but syncope can occur. The right ventricular origin is revealed by a left bundle branch block, right axis deviation morphology during tachycardia (Figure 8.1). Very occasionally the arrhythmia originates from the left ventricular outflow tract. A left ventricular origin is suggested by a right bundle branch block morphology in lead V1 (Figure 8.2). Cases have been recorded in which there are both right and left ventricular outflow tract origins, perhaps indicative of two exit sites from a single origin. During sinus rhythm the ECG and echocardiogram are normal. All other cardiac investigations (signal-averaged ECG, myocardial biopsy, coronary arteriography, left ventricular angiography) are normal and are not usually performed unless there is some specific indication to do so.

Proposed mechanisms

It is characteristic of this form of tachycardia that it can be transiently suppressed (in the case of repetitive extrasystoles) or terminated (in the case of sustained paroxysms) by intravenous adenosine or vagal manoeuvres,

70

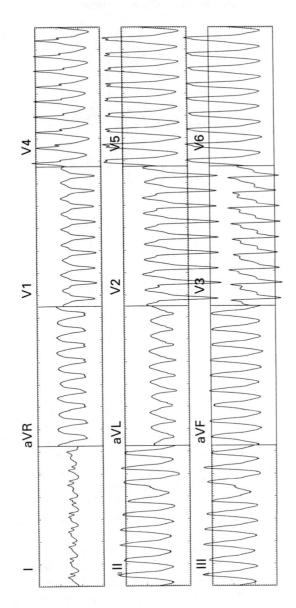

Figure 8.1 12-lead ECG of right ventricular outflow tract tachycardia.

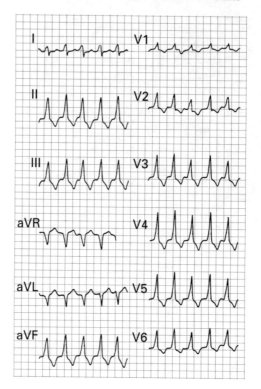

Figure 8.2   12-lead ECG of left ventricular outflow tract tachycardia.

providing support for the suggestion that this arrhythmia is caused by trig-gered activity within individual myocytes. Work on isolated myocytes has shown that stimulation of the beta-adrenergic receptor by catecholamines activates adenylate cyclase and the production of intracellular cAMP. This in turn causes phosphorylation of the L-type Ca^{2+} channel and thereby an increase in intracellular calcium which itself leads to oscillatory release of Ca^{2+} from the sarcoplasmic reticulum and a transient inward current due to Na^+ Ca^{2+} exchange. This transient inward current is associated with the appear-ance of delayed after-depolarisations and triggered activity. Adenosine has no direct electrophysiological effect on ventricular myocardium, but works indi-rectly by inhibiting adenylate cyclase activity and thereby catecholamine-induced stimulation of cAMP (Figure 8.3). Increased vagal tone acts via muscarinic (rather than adenosine) receptors to produce similar effects via inhibition of the same second messenger cascade. Intravenous verapamil is also effective in termination of RVOT tachycardia, consistent with a mecha-nism based on triggered activity secondary to intracellular calcium overload.

Prognosis and treatment

Adenosine-sensitive RVOT tachycardia is not associated with sudden death and is thought to have a normal prognosis. This is in contrast with VTs

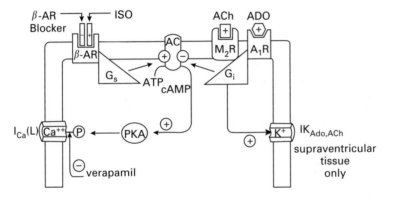

Figure 8.3 The intracellular effects of adenosine receptor stimulation and their relationship with those of vagal stimulation. AC=adenylate cyclase; ACh=acetylcholine; ADO=adenosine; A_1R=adenosine A1 receptor; β-AR=beta adrenergic receptor; ISO=isoproterenol; G_s=stimulatory G protein; G_i=inhibitory G protein; M_2R=muscarinic cholinergic receptor; PKA=protein kinase A. (*From* Lerman *et al.* Mechanism of repetitive monomorphic ventricular tachycardia. *Circulation* 1995;**92**:421–9.)

associated with right ventricular dysplasia, from which it must be distinguished (see Chapter 13). Tachycardias may be controlled by prophylactic verapamil or beta blockade, but ablation of the right (or left) ventricular outflow tract source is usually very successful (90%) and is to be recommended in those with troublesome symptoms.

Left ventricular intrafascicular tachycardia ("fascicular tachycardia")

This is the second most common form of "idiopathic" VT and originates from the region of the left posterior fascicle (posteroapical LV septum).

Clinical presentation, surface ECG, and diagnostic tests

Presentation is usually with palpitations and a paroxysmal sustained VT with a right bundle branch block, left axis deviation morphology (Figure 8.4). More rarely, the arrhythmia arises from the region of the left anterior fascicle (anterosuperior left ventricular septum) leading to a right bundle branch block, right axis deviation pattern during tachycardia. QRS duration is relatively narrow (<140 ms) during VT due to the proximity of the source to the normal conducting system. As with cases of RVOT tachycardia, during sinus rhythm the ECG and echocardiogram are normal. All other cardiac investigations (signal-averaged ECG, myocardial biopsy, coronary arteriography, left ventricular angiography) are normal and are not usually performed unless there is some specific indication to do so.

73

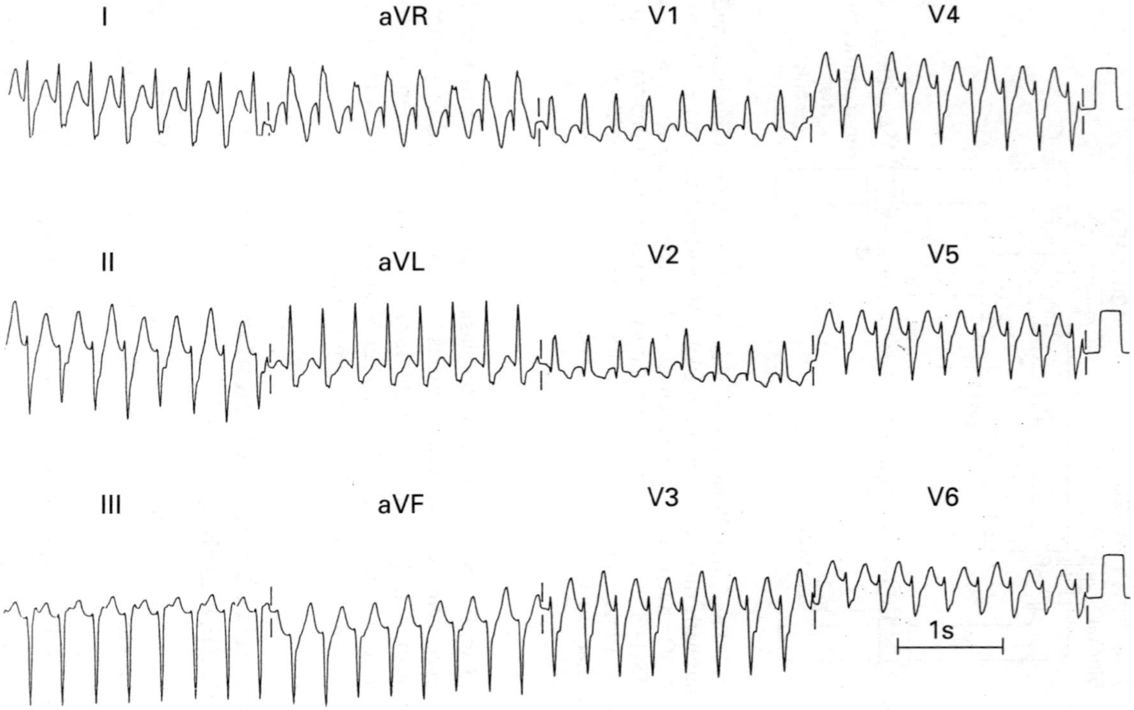

Figure 8.4 12-lead ECG of fascicular tachycardia.

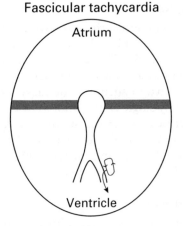

Figure 8.5 Schematic representation of fascicular tachycardia, with site of origin close to the left bundle branch, leading to a relatively narrow, RBBB complex during tachycardia.

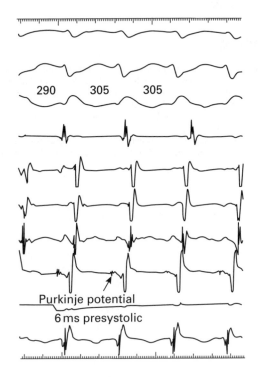

Figure 8.6 "Purkinje potential" preceding ventricular activation recorded at a site of successful catheter ablation of fascicular tachycardia. (*From* Lai *et al*. Entrance site of the slow conduction zone of verapamil-sensitive idiopathic left ventricular tachycardia. *J Cardiovasc Electrophysiol* 1998;**9**:184–90.)

Proposed mechanisms

In contrast to RVOT tachycardia, there is strong evidence to suggest that fascicular tachycardia is caused by a localised re-entrant mechanism either within the Purkinje network (Figure 8.5) or involving a false tendon extending from the posteroinferior left ventricle to the basal septum. The tachycardia is not sensitive to adenosine or vagal manoeuvres and can be initiated or terminated by single extra stimuli. The tachycardia is responsive to verapamil, however, leading to the suggestion that the Purkinje fibres that make up the re-entrant circuit have partially depolarised resting membrane potentials, with depolarising currents more dependent on slow inward Ca^{2+} current than on depressed fast Na^+ channels.

Prognosis and treatment

Fascicular tachycardia is not associated with sudden death and is thought to have a normal prognosis. Tachycardias may be controlled by prophylactic verapamil, but ablation in the posteroapical LV septal region, guided by "Purkinje" potentials (Figure 8.6) and early activation during tachycardia, is usually very successful (90%) and is to be recommended in those with troublesome symptoms.

Further reading

Griffith MJ, Garratt CJ, Rowland E, et al. Effects of intravenous adenosine on verapamil-sensitive "idiopathic" ventricular tachycardia. Am J Cardiol 1994;73:759–64.

Lerman BB, Belardinelli L, West GA, et al. Adenosine-sensitive ventricular tachycardia: evidence suggesting cyclic AMP-mediated triggered activity. Circulation 1986;74:270–80.

Lerman BB, Stein KM, Markowitz SM. Mechanisms of idiopathic left ventricular tachycardia. J Cardiovasc Electrophysiol 1997;8:571–83.

Ohe T, Aihara N, Kamakura S, et al. Long-term outcome of verapamil-sensitive sustained left ventricular tachycardia in patients without structural heart disease. J Am Coll Cardiol 1995;25:54–8.

9: Ventricular tachycardia and fibrillation in the setting of ischaemic heart disease

Definitions

Ventricular tachycardia (VT) is a tachyarrhythmia (more than 3 beats at a rate greater than 100 beats per minute) that originates in the ventricle. Ventricular fibrillation (VF) refers to that form of ventricular tachycardia that is associated with an irregular, continuously varying electrocardiographic pattern and total cessation of cardiac output (see Figure 4.2). In Europe and North America the commonest cause of these arrhythmias is ischaemic heart disease. It is useful to subclassify these arrhythmias into two broad groups:

- Ventricular arrhythmias occurring within 24 hours of acute myocardial infarction (peri-infarction arrhythmias)
- Ventricular arrhythmias occurring after the acute phase of myocardial infarction (scar-related arrhythmias). This group is thought to be caused by the presence of the myocardial scar that develops after myocardial infarction rather than myocardial infarction or ischaemia itself.

Clinical presentation and electrocardiographic characteristics

Peri-infarction ventricular arrhythmias are nearly always *polymorphic*. If they self-terminate they are referred to as polymorphic ventricular tachycardia (Figure 9.1), and if sustained they are referred to as ventricular fibrillation. Of those episodes of VF that occur, approximately 60% occur within 4 hours and 80% within 12 hours of onset of symptoms. The life-threatening nature of this arrhythmia provided the rationale for the development of coronary care units in the 1960s, with facilities for rapid diagnosis and defibrillation. The incidence of VF in the setting of acute myocardial infarction has decreased dramatically in the past decade, probably due to the use of thrombolytic and other therapies such as intravenous beta blockade.

Scar-related arrhythmias are usually regular *monomorphic* ventricular tachycardias (Figure 9.2), although less commonly may take the form of

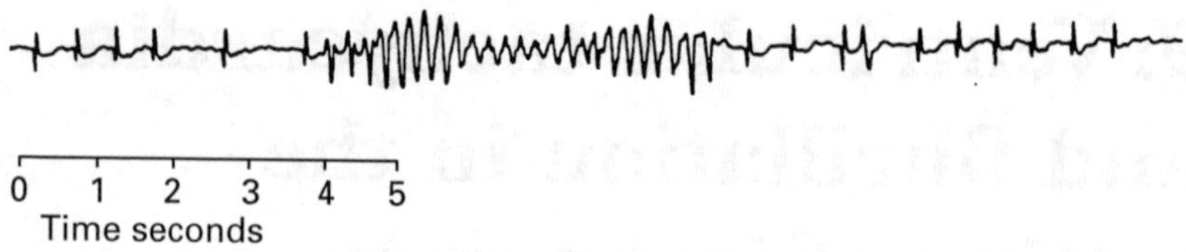

Figure 9.1 Non-sustained polymorphic VT in the setting of acute myocardial infarction. (*From* Clayton RH, Murray A, Higham PD, Campbell RW. Self terminating ventricular tachyarrhythmia – a diagnostic dilemma. *Lancet* 1993;**341**:93–5.

polymorphic VT or VF. Although these arrhythmias occur most commonly in the first three months after infarction, they can occur up to 15 or 20 years later. They may present with regular palpitations, syncope, or shortness of breath. There is usually no obvious precipitating factor and the episodes are usually recurrent, often with weeks or months between episodes. Ventricular tachycardia may self-terminate within a few seconds (non-sustained), continue for hours until appropriately treated (sustained), or alternatively degenerate to VF. Ventricular tachycardias that are very rapid (over 200 beats per minute) are particularly likely to degenerate to VF. Occasionally, scar-related VT can be incessant: this may occur relatively soon after myocardial infarction (approximately 48 hours) or be associated with the use of antiarrhythmic drugs. Incessant VT has a very poor prognosis.

Mechanisms

Acute myocardial ischaemia is known to be associated with a number of potentially arrhythmogenic changes, including shortening of action potential duration, accumulation of extracellular potassium, slowing of conduction velocity, and enhanced sympathetic activity. Ventricular fibrillation itself is thought to be due to functional re-entrant mechanisms, possibly in the form of spiral waves of electrical activity rotating throughout ventricular tissue in a self-sustaining way.

With regard to mechanisms, most of the research performed to date relates to regular (scar-related) VT. In the great majority of cases, this arrhythmia is caused by a macro re-entrant circuit (often extending over several centimetres) sited in the "border zone" at the edge of a myocardial scar and involves slow conduction through surviving myocardial fibres running through the scar. These surviving fibres can be considered as having an exit, where the excitation wave front emerges from the scar and propagates across the ventricles to produce the QRS complex (Figure 9.3). In addition to an exit, the circuit also can be imagined as having a central zone of slow conduction and a proximal region. After the circulating wave front emerges from the exit, it propagates along the border of the infarct region, through an outer loop which may be a broad band of non-infarcted tissue. If there is non-infarcted tissue on both sides of the slow conducting zone then there may be two outer loops, forming a circuit that has been

78

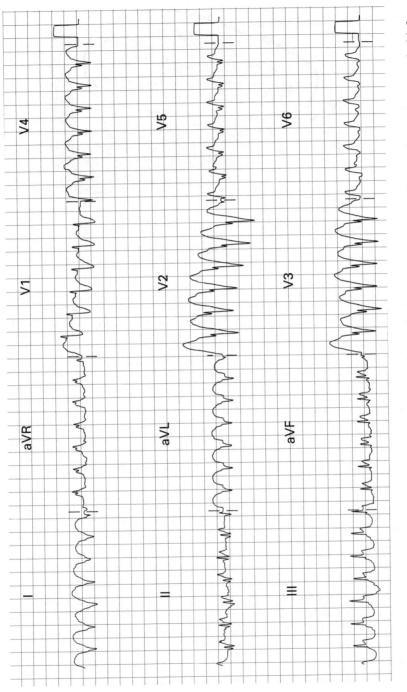

Figure 9.2   Monomorphic VT in the setting of previous myocardial infarction. QRS complexes are wide and do not have a typical left or right bundle branch block pattern.

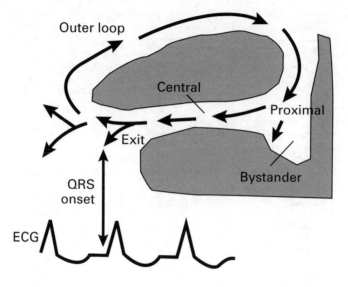

Figure 9.3   Schematic diagram of the postulated re-entry circuit involved in the generation of VT in the setting of previous myocardial infarction. The wavefront propagates through a relatively narrow path in the infarct region (*black arrows*). Depolarisation of the tissue in this path is not detected on the surface ECG: it occurs during the diastolic period. The QRS is inscribed as the excitation wave front emerges from the narrow path and propagates across the ventricles in what is described as an outer loop. This loop is usually broad and a focal ablation lesion in this area is unlikely to abolish the re-entrant activity: the narrow path within infarcted tissue is the region most susceptible to ablation lesions. The individual components of the re-entry circuit can be identified by pacing from a catheter positioned in the region. Pacing in the exit, central, or proximal regions can reset or entrain the VT without altering the QRS morphology and are good potential ablation sites. (*From* Stevenson WG, Friedman PL, Ganz LI. Radio frequency catheter ablation of ventricular tachycardia late after myocardial infarction. *J Cardiovasc Electrophysiol* 1997;**8**:1309–19.)

described as a "figure of 8" (Figure 9.4). Although such re-entrant circuits are often described as functional (in that there may be regions of conduction block during tachycardia in myocardial tissue that conducts during sinus rhythm), they are usually fixed anatomically. It is likely that the circuitry is much more complicated than this model in many cases of clinical VT, with two or more areas of slow conduction that may interact in different ways. The details of the re-entrant pathways in VT are very important in terms of catheter ablation treatment (see later).

Prognosis

The occurrence of VF in the setting of acute myocardial infarction is obviously a life-threatening event but, of those patients that survive defibrillation of VF to hospital discharge, one-year mortality is not increased over patients with uncomplicated infarcts.

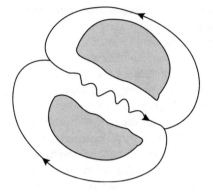

Figure 9.4   Figure-of-8 re-entry. This well-known stylised model of re-entrant activity underlying VT differs from that in Figure 9.3 only in the sense that there are two "outer loops" as opposed to one.

The prognosis of patients with scar-related monomorphic VT is based on three factors.

- *Clinical history*: Patients presenting with poorly tolerated ventricular tachycardia (low blood pressure or syncope) have a much poorer prognosis following acute termination than patients with well-tolerated ventricular tachycardia.
- *Ventricular function*: Patients with poor ventricular function have a poorer prognosis than those with good ventricular function.
- *Inducibility of ventricular tachycardia at electrophysiology study*: Patients with rapid ventricular arrhythmia inducible at electrophysiology study have a poorer prognosis than those who do not, particularly if such rapid arrhythmias cannot be rendered non-inducible by drug treatment.

Patients with poorly tolerated ventricular tachycardia, poor ventricular function, and inducible rapid ventricular tachycardia at electrophysiology study have an approximately 50% one-year survival. Mode of death in these patients is either by degeneration of ventricular tachycardia to ventricular fibrillation or the development of progressive heart failure.

Investigations

The diagnosis of ventricular fibrillation requires only an electrocardiogram and a clinical examination. Ventricular tachycardia is usually diagnosed from a combination of history (previous myocardial infarction), examination (evidence of dissociation of ventricular and atrial activity, such as cannon A waves in the neck), and surface electrocardiographic findings (see Chapter 15).

Coronary arteriography is indicated in patients with sustained ventricular tachycardia in the setting of previous myocardial infarction as well as those thought to have critical ischaemia, as it is often the severity of the underlying ischaemic heart disease that determines the prognosis and appropriate management in this patient group (see later). Echocardiography is usually performed for the same reasons.

Electrophysiology study may be indicated for either diagnostic or prognostic reasons. Ventricular tachycardia may not have been documented by surface electrocardiography, or the diagnosis may not be absolutely certain from the electrocardiogram (Chapter 15). Diagnosis of ventricular tachycardia at electrophysiology study requires the demonstration of a rapid ventricular rate that is dissociated from atrial activity. Ventricular tachycardia can be induced in over 90% of patients who experience spontaneous episodes of ventricular tachycardia (Figure 9.5). Ventricular tachycardia cannot be induced in normal individuals. Ventricular fibrillation (or ventricular flutter) on the other hand can be induced in normal individuals if the stimulation protocol is sufficiently aggressive and as a consequence this finding at electrophysiology study may be a non-specific response (Figure 9.6).

It has been shown by a number of researchers that inducibility of ventricular tachycardia at electrophysiology study is associated with a relatively poor prognosis (see below), particularly if the induced ventricular tachycardia is rapid and cannot be slowed or rendered non-inducible by the infusion of an antiarrhythmic drug. Until recently, electrophysiology studies were also used to guide drug therapy. Patients would be started on a particular drug and then ventricular tachycardia stimulation attempted. If ventricular tachycardia was not inducible then patients would be discharged on this particular drug treatment. There is now a considerable controversy about the value of such a strategy and currently electrophysiology studies are rarely performed for this purpose.

Treatment

Patients with ventricular fibrillation in the setting of *acute myocardial infarction* should be managed in the conventional way (beta blockade, thrombolysis, aspirin, ACE inhibitors) following defibrillation. Previously it has been suggested that frequent ventricular premature beats, early coupling (the "R on T" phenomenon), or salvoes in the setting of acute myocardial infarction were "warning" arrhythmias that precede polymorphic VT and VF. It is now clear, however, that such arrhythmias are present in as many uncomplicated infarctions as in infarctions complicated by VF. As a consequence, prophylactic treatment of these arrhythmias, for instance with lidocaine, is no longer recommended. In fact there is a trend towards increased mortality in trials where this treatment has been given. There is an association between hypokalaemia and the risk of VF in the coronary care unit and it is likely that correction of these abnormalities may prevent some episodes. If VF does occur and is recurrent it is thought that administration of intravenous bretylium, magnesium, or amiodarone may be helpful.

After recovery these patients (in common with patients with uncomplicated infarctions) should undergo investigation to detect the presence of reversible ischaemia, using either exercise electrocardiography or radionuclide perfusion

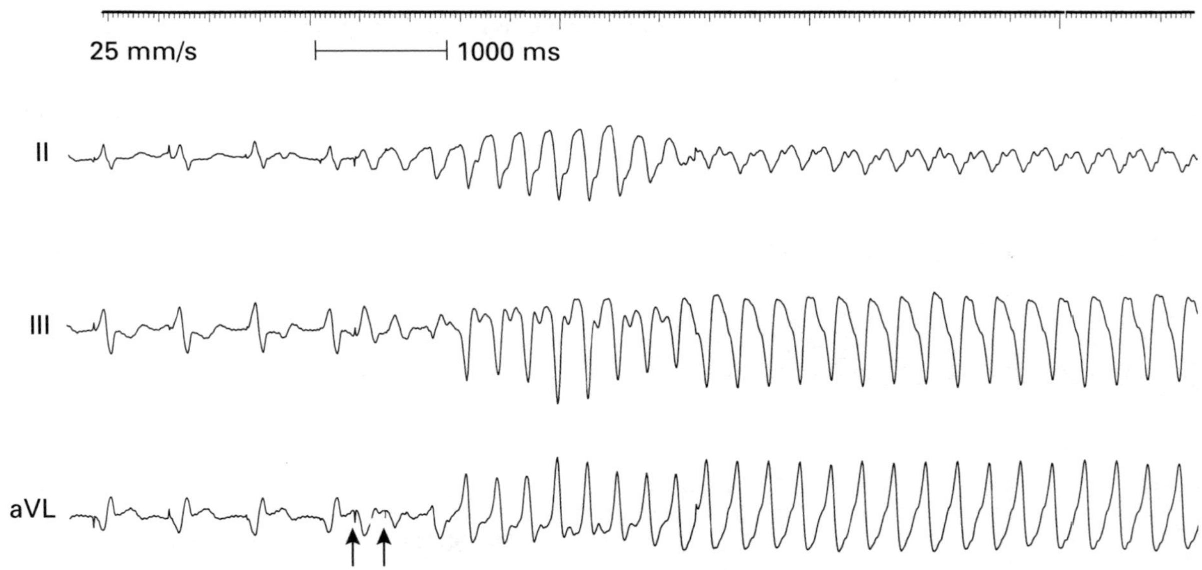

Figure 9.5 Stimulation of a monomorphic VT by two ventricular extrastimuli (arrows) at electrophysiology study. Intially the VT looks polymorphic before stabilising to a monomorphic pattern.

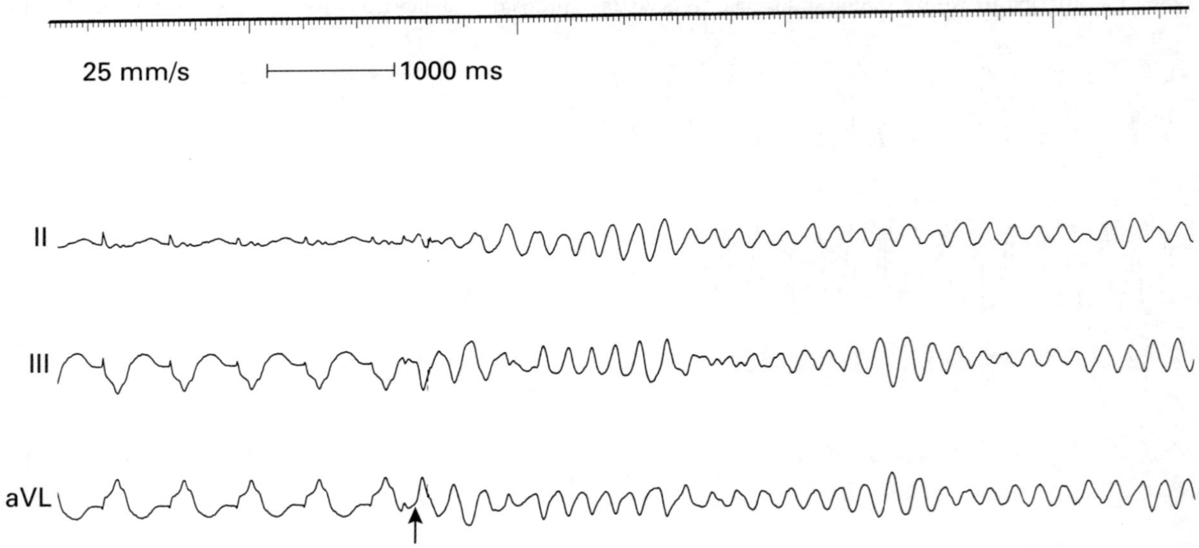

25 mm/s

1000 ms

II

III

aVL

Figure 9.6 Induction of VF at electrophysiology study by a single extra stimulus (arrow).

imaging with pharmacological stress. Specific investigations designed to identify those post-infarction patients at risk of sudden death include echocardiography, ambulatory ECG monitoring, and heart rate variability assessment: in many centres such tests are not performed routinely but are becoming increasingly relevant with the publication of implantable cardioverter trials such as MADIT (Multicentre Automatic Defibrillator Implantation Trial) (see Chapter 18). As stated previously, the prognosis of acute myocardial infarction patients surviving peri-infarction VF is no different from those with uncomplicated infarcts; consequently post-infarct assessment is the same whether peri-infarction VF occurred or not.

Patients with *recurrent monomorphic VT* can be treated in a number of different ways.

Drugs

The most commonly used drugs for the management of recurrent VT are amiodarone and beta blockade. In the CASCADE trial (Cardiac Arrest in Seattle: Conventional versus Amiodarone Drug Evaluation), survivors of cardiac arrest were randomised to receive either empiric treatment with amiodarone or treatment with conventional (usually class I) antiarrhythmic drugs guided by electrophysiologic testing, Holter monitoring, or both. Electrophysiologic testing involves determining the effect of particular antiarrhythmic drugs on VT inducibility at electrophysiologic study. Low dose empiric amiodarone was significantly better at reducing the incidence of cardiac mortality and recurrent arrhythmic events. Beta blockade has been shown to improve prognosis following myocardial infarction. Sotalol when used in relatively high dosage combines an amiodarone-like effect together with beta blockade and has been shown to reduce the recurrence of ventricular tachycardia in patients with implanted defibrillators in a randomised trial. Class I antiarrhythmic drugs such as quinidine and flecainide are used much less often nowadays in view of their known risk of proarrhythmic effects and increased mortality of patients with ischaemic heart disease. The problem with the use of antiarrhythmic drugs in patients with ventricular tachycardia is that it is difficult to predict who will respond and who will not. As the first recurrence of ventricular tachycardia may be fatal, this is a considerable disadvantage.

Implantable cardioverter defibrillators (see Chapter 18)

To date, implantable cardioverter defibrillators have been shown to confer prognostic benefit in the following patient groups:

- Patients presenting with ventricular fibrillation in the absence of acute myocardial infarction
- Patients presenting with poorly tolerated ventricular tachycardia
- Patients with non-sustained ventricular tachycardia, impaired left ventricular function, and inducible arrhythmias at electrophysiology study that are not suppressed by antiarrhythmic drugs.

These devices also have a role in patients with well-tolerated ventricular tachycardia requiring multiple hospital admissions. They are capable of delivering bursts of ventricular pacing which are able to terminate regular ventricular tachycardia automatically without the requirement for antiarrhythmic drugs or electrical shock.

Radiofrequency catheter ablation

Currently catheter ablation is a relatively uncommon form of therapy for VT. The small lesion size associated with radiofrequency catheter ablation relative to the size of the re-entrant circuits makes precise mapping of the circuit critical for success. As a consequence of the anatomy of the circuits (see Figure 9.3), only lesions delivered within the narrow components of the re-entrant (the central proximal or exit zones) are likely to be successful. Lesions delivered in the broad outer loop are unlikely to terminate tachycardia, particularly if there is more than one such loop (see Figure 9.4). Conventional methods of mapping use endocardial recordings and the response to pacing from the ablation catheter in different sites to define the circuit precisely. This is time-consuming and is only feasible in patients with haemodynamically stable tachycardia. Recently, mapping techniques have become available which can record electrograms from very many sites simultaneously and thus define the crucial components of the circuit during (in theory) a single beat of tachycardia. A particular disadvantage is that although one may be able to ablate a re-entrant circuit causing clinical tachycardia, this is no guarantee that other re-entrant circuits are not present and the risk of subsequent ventricular arrhythmias and sudden death may remain. Catheter ablation can be life-saving, however, for patients with incessant VT and can markedly improve the quality of life for some patients with VTs that are causing frequent shocks from an implantable defibrillator.

Surgery

Surgery has a relatively small role in the management of ventricular tachycardia and fibrillation. Patients with coronary disease should undergo coronary artery bypass grafting if they have left main stem or significant triple vessel disease in the same way as would a patient without ventricular arrhythmias. Most patients with scar-related ventricular arrhythmias will continue to have their arrhythmias after coronary revascularisation surgery. Attempts to remove the substrates for re-entry during these operations (endocardial resection) are successful, but may be associated with further impairment of ventricular function and increased mortality.

Further reading

El-Sherif N. Reentrant mechanisms in ventricular arrhythmias. In: Zipes D and Jalife J eds. *Cardiac electrophysiology from cell to bedside*, 2nd edn. Philadelphia: WB Saunders, 1995.

Josephson ME, Almendral JM, Buxton AE, *et al.* Mechanisms of ventricular tachycardia. *Circulation* 1978;57:431.

Pathmanathan RK, Lau EW, Cooper J, Newton L, Skehan JD, Garratt CJ, Griffith MJ. Potential impact of antiarrhythmic drugs versus implantable defibrillators in the management of ventricular arrhythmias: the Midlands trial of empiric amiodarone versus electrophysiologically guided intervention and cardioverter implant registry data. *Heart* 1998;**80**: 68–70.

Stevenson WG. Catheter mapping of ventricular tachycardia. In: Zipes D and Jalife J eds. *Cardiac electrophysiology from cell to bedside*, 2nd edn. Philadelphia: WB Saunders, 1995.

10: Ventricular tachycardia and fibrillation in the setting of dilated or hypertrophic cardiomyopathy

Although most patients with VT or VF have coronary disease, in some patients these arrhythmias are caused by one of the cardiomyopathies. Because of the relative rarity of these conditions (compared with coronary disease) much less is known about mechanisms and management of ventricular arrhythmias in this setting.

Dilated cardiomyopathy

Dilated cardiomyopathy is a syndrome characterised by dilatation of one or both ventricles and impaired systolic function. Although coronary disease is the most common cause of this syndrome (Chapter 9), this chapter will address the cardiac arrhythmias associated with dilated cardiomyopathy of unknown origin (idiopathic cardiomyopathy or IDC). The incidence of IDC is thought to be approximately 5 cases per 100 000 population.

Clinical presentation

Patients with an acute myocarditic element to their condition (see below) may present with very rapid VT or VF, similar to patients presenting with acute ischaemia/infarction. Unlike the ischaemic equivalent, however, there is no good evidence to suggest that such patients lose their propensity to malignant arrhythmia once the acute episode is over. Ventricular fibrillation and cardiac arrest can also occur in the setting of chronic IDC, although the incidence is unclear. Certainly sudden death is common in IDC, although a percentage of such deaths are due to bradyarrhythmias. Patients may also present with sustained VT, including bundle branch re-entrant tachycardia (see below).

88

Aetiology

At least 20% of patients with this condition have familial disease. In some patients an autoimmune condition is postulated and a further group develop cardiomyopathy following an acute episode of viral myocarditis.

Mechanism of arrhythmia

At autopsy, extensive subendocardial scarring is seen in many patients and, together with multiple patchy areas of replacement fibrosis, this provides a substrate for functional re-entry and VF.

Some patients with IDC experience bundle branch re-entry, producing sustained VT via a macro re-entrant circuit involving the His–Purkinje system, usually with antegrade conduction over the right bundle branch and retrograde conduction over the left bundle branch (Figure 10.1). This arrhythmia is very unusual in the absence of cardiomyopathy, and probably is caused by fibrotic changes within the conducting system sufficient to cause slow conduction and unidirectional block (see Chapter 3).

Diagnosis

Diagnosis of IDC is based on echocardiography and the exclusion of coronary disease by coronary arteriography. Bundle branch re-entrant tachycardia usually has a left bundle branch morphology that is also present in sinus rhythm. Formal diagnosis of this arrhythmia requires electrophysiology study.

Prognosis and assessment of risk

Studies assessing the variables used to predict survival in IDC demonstrate that the severity of left ventricular function is the most consistent predictor of risk for sudden death, and that the presence of complex ventricular arrhythmias on Holter is both very common and of little discriminant value.

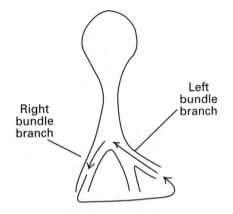

Figure 10.1   Schematic representation of bundle branch re-entrant tachycardia.

There are very little data on the prognostic value of electrophysiology studies in this condition.

Therapy

Bundle branch re-entrant tachycardia is an important arrhythmia to recognise, as catheter ablation of the right bundle branch is curative. Antiarrhythmic drugs are not normally successful in this form of tachycardia. The mainstay of treatment of dilated cardiomyopathy is that of heart failure of any underlying condition. ACE inhibitors and beta blockers are of value in improving prognosis in patients with IDC and there is some evidence that amiodarone may also be of some value in those with ventricular arrhythmias. In those patients who have already suffered VF, an ICD is indicated (see Chapter 18). Cardiac transplant is appropriate in selected cases.

Hypertrophic cardiomyopathy

The prevalence of hypertrophic cardiomyopathy (HCM) is now thought to be as high as 1 in 500 individuals, but many of these remain asymptomatic or minimally symptomatic throughout their lives. Excellent reviews on the management of HCM are available (see Further Reading) and this chapter is restricted to mechanisms and management of the cardiac arrhythmias associated with the condition.

Clinical presentation

From the cardiac arrhythmia point of view, the main forms of presentation are those of atrial fibrillation, non-sustained VT, and VF/sudden cardiac death. Much of the investigational effort invested in patients with HCM is undertaken in order to determine risk of the latter complication. In contrast to patients with ischaemic heart disease, IDC, and RV dysplasia, presentation with sustained monomorphic VT is rare.

Aetiology

Hypertrophic cardiomyopathy is a genetic disease of the sarcomere and is caused by a mutation in any one of the genes encoding sarcomeric proteins, i.e. beta-myosin heavy chains, cardiac troponin T, alpha-tropomyosin, myosin-binding protein, or myosin light chains (see Further Reading).

Diagnosis

The clinical diagnosis of HCM is made on the basis of 2D echocardiographic evidence of a hypertrophied but non-dilated left ventricle in the absence of other cardiac or systemic disease (principally hypertension) to account for the hypertrophy. Genetic markers are useful diagnostically in families in which the relevant mutation is known but the number of identified mutations in HCM is such that this approach is of very limited use in sporadic cases.

Mechanism of arrhythmia

The characteristic cardiac histological finding in patients with HCM is the presence of myocyte and myofibrillar disarray surrounding areas of increased loose connective tissue, thought to be a maladaptive response to impaired sarcomere function. A number of studies have shown that the degree of disarray is related to risk of death; the disorganised myocyte structure is likely to act as a substrate for inhomogenous and slow conduction within the ventricle, predisposing to functional re-entry and VF.

Prognosis and assessment of risk

The major complication of the disease is the occurrence of sudden death. The principal risk factors for sudden death are a history of syncope, a family history of sudden death, the presence of non-sustained VT on Holter, and extreme hypertrophy (LV wall thickness of at least 3 cm). These factors are sensitive but not specific for the risk of death, i.e. although patients without these risk factors are definitely at low risk, a high proportion of those in whom one or more factors are present will not die suddenly. Standard electrophysiology study/ventricular stimulation protocols are probably of no value in the assessment of risk, although there may be a future role for more novel electrophysiological assessments aimed at detecting inhomogenous and slow conduction within the ventricle. There has been much debate about the mechanism of sudden death in HCM, but a recent large retrospective study of patients with implanted cardioverter defibrillators has revealed that sudden death is aborted in patients with ICDs. In this study there were deaths in only two out of 128 patients (due to severe systolic dysfunction), strongly supporting the suggestion that rapid VT/VF is the principal cause of sudden death in HCM (Figure 10.2). Appropriate defibrillator shocks (rapid VT/VF documented by means of electrograms stored in the ICD) occurred at a rate of 11% a year in patients with previous episodes of cardiac arrest (secondary prevention) and 5% per

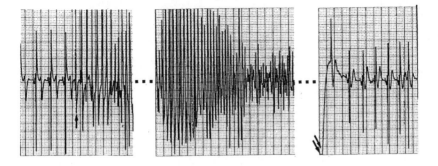

Figure 10.2   Recording from an ICD implanted in a 30-year-old patient with HCM showing onset of VT/VF and defibrillator shock (*double arrow*) restoring sinus rhythm. (*From* Maron BJ, Casey SA, Almquist AK. Aborted sudden cardiac death in hypertrophic cardiomyopathy. *J Cardiovasc Electrophysiol* 1999;**10**:263.)

year in those with no such previous events (primary prevention) but with other clinical risk factors (see above).

Therapy

There is a very strong case to be made for implantation of an ICD in those patients with a previous episode of cardiac arrest and in those thought to be at very high risk on the basis of clinical criteria. There are non-randomised data suggesting amiodarone may also lower risk, but in the study of ICDs discussed above a third of those patients in whom sudden death was aborted by defibrillator shocks were already taking amiodarone. It should be remembered that the mechanism of sudden death in some patients may be related to rapidly conducted AF, coexistent accessory pathways, or conduction system disease and these possibilities should also be considered and treated on an individual patient basis.

Further reading

Caceres J, Jazayeri M, McKinnie J, *et al.* Sustained bundle branch reentry as a mechanism of clinical tachycardia. *Circulation* 1989;**79**:256–70.

Cohen TJ, Chien WW, Lurie KG, *et al.* Radiofrequency catheter ablation for treatment of bundle branch reentrant ventricular tachycardia: results and long term follow up. *J Am Coll Cardiol* 1991;**18**:1767–73.

Maron BJ, Shen WK, Link MS, *et al.* Efficacy of implantable cardioverter defibrillators for the prevention of sudden death in patients with hypertrophic cardiomyopathy. *N Engl J Med* 2000;**342**:365–73.

Spirito P, Seidman CE, McKenna WJ, Baron BJ. The management of hypertrophic cardiomyopathy. *N Engl J Med* 1997;**336**:775–85.

11: Ventricular fibrillation in the setting of a structurally normal heart

It is estimated that perhaps 4–5% of patients suffering cardiac arrest due to ventricular fibrillation have no evidence of structural heart disease or identifiable reversible cause for their arrhythmia. These patients are frequently young (20s, 30s) and are often considered as having "primary electrical disease". A number of studies have indicated that risk of recurrence of VF after resuscitation in these patients is high – in the order of 20–30% over the next three years. Recently some of these patients have been identified as having a familial VF syndrome referred to as the *Brugada syndrome*.

Clinical presentation and electrocardiographic findings

The Brugada syndrome is characterised by ST segment elevation in leads V1–3 in sinus rhythm, often but not always accompanied by apparent right bundle branch block. The syndrome is familial (autosomal dominant with variable expression) and is particularly common in Southeast Asia, where it is a leading cause of sudden death in young men. In this latter group a characteristic feature is that death occurs suddenly with a groan, usually during sleep, late at night. The frequency of this syndrome in the overall "idiopathic VF" population is difficult to ascertain, as the typical ECG changes may be intermittent, or only revealed after the infusion of Na^+-channel blocking drugs (Figure 11.1).

Pathology

There is no evidence of histopathological abnormality in the Brugada syndrome or in other forms of idiopathic VF. The characteristic features of arrhythmogenic right ventricular dysplasia are absent. Although some authors have suggested that the two diseases are linked, there is little good evidence for this and their underlying genetic bases are completely different.

Underlying molecular and cellular mechanisms

The finding of ST elevation in the right chest leads is observed in several experimental settings, and cellular studies have suggested that the ECG abnormality in this syndrome may be caused by a marked difference between action potential duration of endocardial and epicardial cells in the

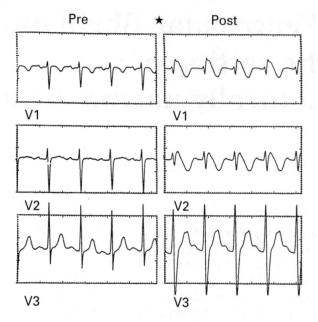

Figure 11.1 Right precordial surface ECG leads before and after infusion of a Na$^+$-channel blocking drug in a patient with the intermittent form of the Brugada syndrome. (*From* Schimizu W, Antzelevitch C, Suyama K *et al*. Effect of sodium channel blockers on ST segment, QRS duration and corrected QT interval in patients with the Brugada syndrome. *J Cardiovasc Electrophysiol* 2000;**11**:1320–9.)

right ventricle. Under certain conditions an increase in net outward current at the end of phase 1 of the action potential can lead to sudden loss of the plateau phase in epicardial cells and marked action potential shortening. Such conditions include an increase in outward I_{TO} or a decrease in inward $I_{Ca^{2+}}$ or I_{Na^+}, for instance associated with use of Na$^+$-channel blocking drugs. This shortening occurs only in epicardial cells and the resultant difference between epicardial/endocardial action potential duration provides both an explanation for the ECG pattern and a substrate for re-entrant activity that may underlie ventricular fibrillation (Figure 11.2).

Altered function of I_{TO}, $I_{Ca^{2+}}$ or I_{Na^+} are possible mechanisms for the Brugada syndrome, and to date several mutations in the sodium channel gene SCN5A have been identified in affected families. These include a missense mutation in the extracellular loop between transmembrane segments S3 and S4 of domain IV, a 2-nucleotide insertion that disrupts the splice–donor sequence of intron 7, and a single nucleotide deletion resulting in an in-frame stop codon which eliminates DIIIS6, DIVS1–DIVS6, and the cardoxy-terminus of SCN5A (Figure 11.3). Unlike LQT mutations on this gene (which lead to gain of function – see Chapter 12), these mutations result in partial loss of function of the Na$^+$ channel, in keeping with the cellular explanation of the ECG findings given above. Further recent work has shown that other families exist without any mutations in

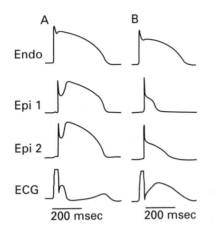

Figure 11.2 Proposed mechanism of ECG changes and arrhythmogenesis in the Brugada syndrome. The two panels show transmembrane action potentials simultaneously recorded from one endocardial and two epicardial sites in an arterially perfused wedge of canine right ventricular tissue. Infusion of the K channel opener pinacidil (panel B) results in selective loss of the plateau phase (dome) in the epicardium and an elevated ST segment on the accompanying ECG. The resultant increase in dispersion of refractoriness provides a substrate for re-entry. (*From* Yan GX, Antzelevitch C. Cellular basis for the Brugada syndrome and other mechanisms of arrhythmogenesis associated with ST segment elevation. *Circulation* 1999;**100**:1660–6.)

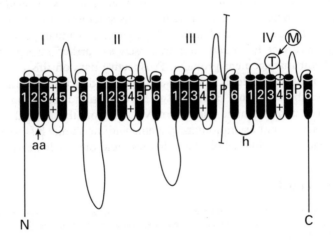

Figure 11.3 Anomalies of Na^+ channel structure identified in patients with Brugada syndrome. Three types of mutations are shown: one missense mutation causing substitution of a highly conserved threonine by methionine in the extracellular loop between transmembrane segments S3 and S4 of domain IV, a 2-nucleotide insertion (AA) that disrupts the splice–donor sequence of intron 7 of SCN5A, and a single nucleotide deletion that results in an in-frame stop codon that eliminates DIIIS6, DIVS1–DIVS6, and the carboxy-terminus of SCN5A.

SCN5A, suggesting that the underlying abnormality may be found in other ion channels in these patients.

Arrhythmia mechanism

As discussed above, there is evidence that the ECG pattern of the Brugada syndrome is caused by a marked disparity between epicardial and endocardial action potentials within the right ventricle. Such dispersion of repolarisation provides an ideal substrate for functional re-entry and generation of VF.

Diagnosis

Patients resuscitated from VF outside the setting of acute myocardial infarction should undergo echocardiography and cardiac catheterisation to exclude underlying structural causes (coronary disease, dilated or hypertrophic cardiomyopathies, right ventricular dysplasia). "Primary electrical disease" is a diagnosis of exclusion but a positive diagnosis of the Brugada syndrome can be made in the presence of the characteristic ECG changes. Flecainide infusion may be appropriate as a diagnostic test in those cases of idiopathic VF with a normal ECG, but should be performed in hospital as this test has been known to induce VF in affected individuals.

Prognosis and treatment

Patients presenting with VF in the absence of structural heart disease (whether they have the Brugada surface ECG pattern or not) have a high risk of recurrence, at a rate of approximately 10% per year. There is no evidence that antiarrhythmic drugs are of any benefit in this situation and implantation of an ICD is to be recommended in all such patients. Individuals presenting with the Brugada surface ECG pattern in the absence of arrhythmias pose a much more difficult management problem. Prospective data on this population is currently being collected but at present firm guidance regarding the best approach to these patients cannot be given. Current advice is to implant an ICD in those asymptomatic relatives of VF survivors that have the Brugada ECG pattern but not asymptomatic patients with no family history of VF or sudden death. Na^+-channel blocking drugs should obviously be avoided.

Further reading

Brugada P, Brugada J. Right bundle branch block, persistent ST segment elevation and sudden cardiac death: a distinct clinical and electrocardiographic syndrome. *J Am Coll Cardiol* 1992;**20**:1391–6.

Brugada R, Brugada J, Antzelevitch C *et al*. Sodium channel blockers identify risk for sudden death in patients with ST segment elevation and right bundle branch block but structurally normal hearts. *Circulation* 2000;**101**:510–15.

Chen Q, Kirsch GE, Zhang D *et al*. Genetic basis and molecular mechanisms for idiopathic ventricular fibrillation. *Nature* 1998;**392**:293–6.

Wever EFD, Hauer RNW, Oomen A, Peters RHJ, Bakker PFA, Robles de Medina EO. Unfavorable outcome in patients with primary electrical disease who survived an episode of ventricular fibrillation. *Circulation* 1993;**88**:1021–9.

12: The congenital long QT syndrome

This dramatic familial syndrome is an important cause of sudden death in children and adolescents and one about which much is known in terms of the fundamental molecular abnormalities.

Clinical presentation

The classical clinical presentation of the condition is with syncope or cardiac arrest in a child or adolescent, often precipitated by emotional or physical stress, associated with a prolonged QT interval on the surface electrocardiogram. The relatively frequent occurrence of convulsions often leads to the misdiagnosis of epilepsy.

Two variants were identified initially: the original syndrome described by Jervell and Lange-Nielson with congenital deafness (autosomal recessive), and the more common Romano–Ward syndrome with normal hearing and autosomal dominant inheritance. Approximately 25% of cases have no evidence of familial involvement.

Pathology and pathophysiology

There are no gross pathological or histopathological abnormalities that have been identified in patients with the syndrome. Until the discovery of the underlying molecular mechanisms involved in the syndrome, the most widely supported mechanistic hypothesis was that of sympathetic imbalance, with relative overactivity of the left-sided cardiac sympathetic nerves. This idea was based on experimental studies involving stimulation and ablation of stellate ganglia and on the improvement of some patients following left cardiac sympathetic denervation (see below). The current view is that sympathetic activity (imbalanced or otherwise) may act as a trigger for arrhythmia generation but the fundamental abnormality in the syndrome is clearly a genetically determined abnormality in ion channel function leading to prolonged repolarisation in ventricular myocytes.

Underlying molecular mechanisms and subclassification based on genotype

The discovery of the first three genes responsible for the long QT syndrome(s) was reported in 1995 and 1996: on chromosome 11 (LQT1), on

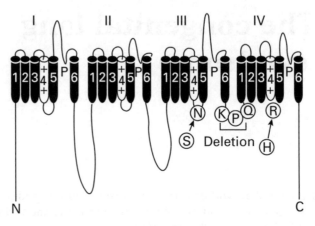

Figure 12.1 Anomalies of Na$^+$ channel structure identified in patients with LQT3. Three types of mutations (one 9 base pair intragenic deletion, and 2 missense mutations) are shown.

chromosome 9 (LQT2), and on chromosome 3 (LQT3). The gene for LQT1 is KvLQT1 which, when coexpressed with minK subunits, produces the I_{Ks} current. Abnormalities in this gene have been found responsible for the recessive Jervell Lange-Nielson syndrome. The gene for LQT2 is HERG, the potassium channel that carries the I_{Kr} current. The gene for LQT3 is SCN5A, the cardiac sodium channel gene (Figure 12.1). Expression of mutant HERG genes results in a decrease in numbers of channels carrying I_{Kr} with a consequent prolongation of action potential duration. Expression of the mutant SCN5A genes has shown that they produce a gain of function, resulting in a small, sustained inward current which is (by a means that is unclear) sufficient to prolong action potentials.

Electrocardiographic findings

The syncopal episodes are due to torsade de pointes (polymorphic VT in the setting of a long QT interval) (Figure 12.2); this form of VT is often self-terminating but there is a high incidence of sudden death in untreated symptomatic individuals due to continuing arrhythmia and VF. Torsade de pointes may be precipitated by a pause (often following a ventricular premature beat) or may occur without precipitating electrocardiographic changes.

Typically the corrected QT interval is above 440 ms in males, 460 ms in females. The extent of QT prolongation is variable and not strictly correlated with the likelihood of syncopal episodes, although values over 600 ms are associated with a high incidence of malignant arrhythmias. About 5% of affected individuals with syncope have a normal QT interval.

Alternation of the T wave (T wave alternans), in polarity or amplitude, may precede torsade de pointes and is a risk factor for malignant arrhythmias.

The three different groups of mutations produce different electrocardiographic phenotypes, seen predominantly in the shape of the T wave

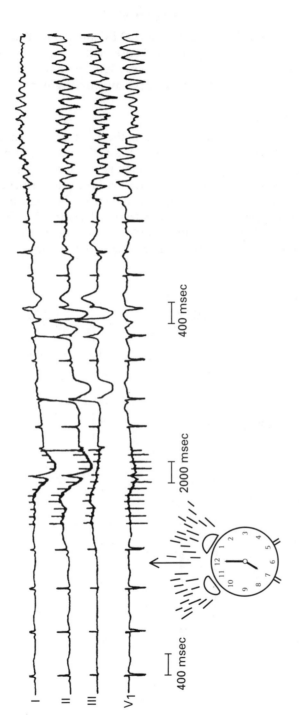

Figure 12.2 Tracings of a 14 year old girl with the long QT syndrome. This patient had a history of losing consciousness after being awakened by thunder or the noise of an alarm clock. Initiation of ventricular fibrillation following an auditory stimulus (alarm clock) is shown. The middle part of the tracing is at a slower paper speed than the beginning and end of the tracing. This patient was treated with beta blockers and remained free of episodes for several years until her boyfriend convinced her that she did not need medications. She interrupted her therapy and died suddenly within a few weeks. Ventricular fibrillation occurring on arousal from sleep by auditory stimuli. (*From* Wellens HJJ, Vermeulen A, Durrer D. *Circulation* 1972;**46**:661–5.)

(Figure 12.3). The T wave is broadest with KvLQT1 mutations, T wave amplitude is lowest in the HERG mutations, and onset of the T wave is most delayed in patients with sodium channel mutations. Although these features hold true in general, there is considerable overlap between the groups.

Arrhythmia mechanisms

Despite over two decades of detailed investigation, the exact mechanism of polymorphic VT in a setting of the congenital long QT syndrome is not known for certain. A number of lines of investigation have shown that there is an increased dispersion of ventricular repolarisation in affected patients, due to particularly prolonged repolarisation in some areas. This may be a substrate for functional determined re-entrant waves of electrical activation, possibly in the form of spirals drifting rapidly through the ventricles. An alternative hypothesis is that early or late after-depolarisations may

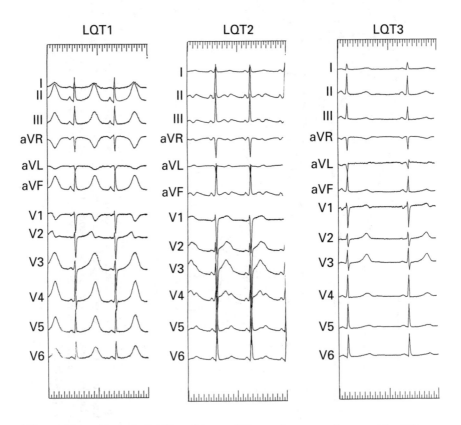

Figure 12.3 Typical ECGs of long QT syndrome patients with different genotypes (see text for description). (*From* Moss AJ, Zareba W, Benhorin J *et al.* ECG T wave patterns in genetically distinct forms of the hereditary long QT syndrome. *Circulation* 1995;**92**:229–34.)

occur and lead to VT as a consequence of triggered activity. There is *in vitro* evidence that ventricular myocytes subjected to beta-adrenergic stimulation develop both types of after-depolarisations over a range of pacing frequencies.

Diagnosis

As in other conditions where diagnosis can be difficult, a "diagnostic score" system is used (Table 12.1). The point score is arbitrarily divided into three categories: less than 2 points = low probability, 2 to 3 points = intermediate probability, 4 points = high probability. This system remains the best means of diagnosis except for those individuals who are relatives of proven cases with a defined abnormal nucleotide sequence. At present molecular diagnosis is limited by the genetic heterogeneity of the syndrome.

Table 12.1   Diagnostic criteria in long QT syndrome.

	Points
Electrocardiographic findings[a]	
QTc[b]	
>480 ms	3
460–470 ms	2
450 (male) ms	1
Torsade de pointes[c]	2
T wave alternans	1
Notched T wave in three leads	1
Low heart rate for age[d]	0·5
Clinical history	
Syncope[c]	
With stress	2
Without stress	1
Congenital deafness	0·5
Family history[e]	
Family members with definite LQTS[f]	1
Unexplained sudden cardiac death below age 30 among immediate family members	0·5

[a]In the absence of medications or disorders known to affect these electrocardiographic features.
[b]QTc calculated by Bazett's formula where QTc = $QT\sqrt{RR}$.
[c]Mutually exclusive.
[d]Resting heart rate below the 2nd percentile for age.
[e]The same family member cannot be counted in both groups.
[f]Definite LQTS is defined by an LQTS score >4.

Scoring: <2 points   = low probability of LQTS
2 to 3 points = intermediate probability of LQTS
>4 points   = high probability of LQTS

(*From* Schwartz PJ, Moss AJ, Vincent GM, Crampton RS. Diagnostic criteria for the long QT syndrome: an update. *Circulation* 1993;**88**:782–4.)

Prognosis

Mortality rate is high in untreated patients after their first episode of syncope, with a 20% incidence of sudden death in the first year and 50% of patients are dead at 15 year follow-up. Consequently all symptomatic patients should receive treatment.

Prognostic assessment and consequent decisions regarding treatment for asymptomatic but affected relatives of long QT syndrome patients are difficult. Schwartz has recommended therapy under six specific circumstances:

- In those with congenital deafness, because risk of a cardiac event is particularly high
- In neonates and for the first year of life because of their enhanced risk during this period
- In siblings and children of those who have already died from the condition
- In those with T wave alternans
- In those where QTc exceeds 600 ms
- When there is ongoing anxiety and request for therapy despite full discussion of the condition.

Therapy

Beta blockade is the mainstay of treatment in the long QT syndrome. Propranolol is the most widely used drug, at a daily dosage of 2–3 mg/kg. Although there are no placebo controlled trials of beta-blocker therapy (and now never will be), treatment of symptomatic patients with beta blockade is associated with marked reduction in mortality (see Figure 12.4).

Left cardiac sympathetic denervation involves the surgical removal of the lower half of the left stellate ganglion (not the upper half to avoid Horner's syndrome) and the first four or five thoracic ganglia. This is done under general anaesthetic and takes approximately 45 minutes. It results in loss of sweating on the left hand, possibly the left forehead, and a mild ptosis. In uncontrolled studies this procedure has produced impressive reductions in cardiac events in patients unresponsive to beta blockade.

Cardiac pacing is indicated if there is evidence of pause-related VT or the use of beta blockade is limited by sinus bradycardia. Cardiac pacing has shown improvement in symptoms in uncontrolled trials but this may relate more to increased beta-blocker use than to any other effect.

Implantable cardioverter defibrillators (ICDs) are indicated in those patients with syncope despite the use of the above therapies, or those affected individuals with a family history of sudden death. Potential problems with the use of these devices in this population include psychological disturbances in adolescents due to repeated ICD discharge for episodes that may well have terminated spontaneously and the requirement for multiple device and lead changes over a lifetime of therapy.

Gene-specific therapies are investigational at present. The sodium-channel blocker mexiletine produces a considerable shortening of the QT interval

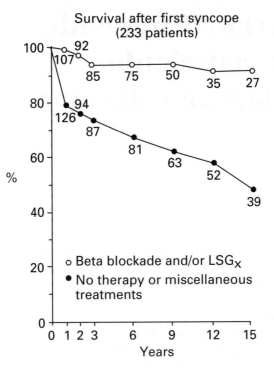

Figure 12.4   Difference between survival of long QT syndrome patients taking beta blockade and those not taking beta blockade in a retrospective study. (*From* Schwartz PJ, Locati E. The idiopathic long QT syndrome: pathogenetic mechanisms and therapy. *Eur Heart J* 1985;6:103–14.)

in LQT3 patients in particular but the clinical benefit of this therapy remains unknown. Similarly, potassium-channel openers may have a beneficial role in LQT2 patients but clinical results are awaited.

Further reading

Curran ME, Splawski I, Timothy KW, *et al.* A molecular basis for cardiac arrhythmia: HERG mutations cause long QT syndrome. *Cell* 1995;80:795–803.

Moss AJ, Zareba W, Benhorin J, *et al.* ECG T wave patterns in genetically distinct forms of the hereditary long QT syndrome. *Circulation* 1995;92:2929–34.

Schwartz PJ. *The congenital long QT syndrome.* New York: Futura Publishing, 1997.

Schwartz PJ, Moss AJ, Vincent GM, Crampton RS. Diagnostic criteria for the long QT syndrome: an update. *Circulation* 1993;88:782–4.

Wang Q, Chen J, Splawski I, *et al.* SCN5A mutations associated with an inherited cardiac arrhythmia, long QT syndrome. *Cell* 1995;80:805–11.

Wang Q, Curran ME, Splawski I, *et al.* Positional cloning of a novel potassium gene: KvLQT1 mutations cause cardiac arrhythmias. *Nature Genetics* 1996;12:17–23.

13: Arrhythmogenic right ventricular dysplasia/cardiomyopathy

Definition

Arrhythmogenic right ventricular cardiomyopathy/dysplasia (ARVD) is a cardiomyopathy predominantly involving the myocardium of the right ventricle which is replaced by fatty or fibro-fatty tissue.

Background

The first important description of the condition was published in 1982 by Marcus and coworkers who reported 24 adult patients with sustained ventricular tachycardia with a left bundle branch block morphology and dilatation of the right ventricle. The potential importance of this condition was highlighted by a necropsy study in 1988 in which it was revealed that 20% of patients under the age of 35 years dying suddenly and unexpectedly in northern Italy had histological findings consistent with arrhythmogenic right ventricular dysplasia. Although this high incidence has subsequently been shown to be somewhat atypical, it has become clear that this condition is often overlooked as a cause of sudden cardiac death in young or middle aged individuals.

Clinical features

In the classical form, the disease presents between the ages of 10 and 40. The symptoms are those of palpitation, presyncope or syncope, which are often exercise-induced in subjects generally considered normal on physical examination. In over half of the patients dying suddenly in the Italian series, death occurred during effort.

The electrocardiogram at rest shows negative T waves in the precordial leads V1 to V5 (Figure 13.1), incomplete right bundle branch block or prolongation of QRS duration greater than 0.12 seconds in leads V1 to V2. Occasionally distinct waves occur after the end of the QRS complex suggesting delayed activation of some portion of the right ventricular wall ("epsilon wave"). The electrocardiogram during symptoms demonstrates the presence of sustained monomorphic ventricular tachycardia with a left bundle branch block pattern or bursts of ventricular ectopic activity.

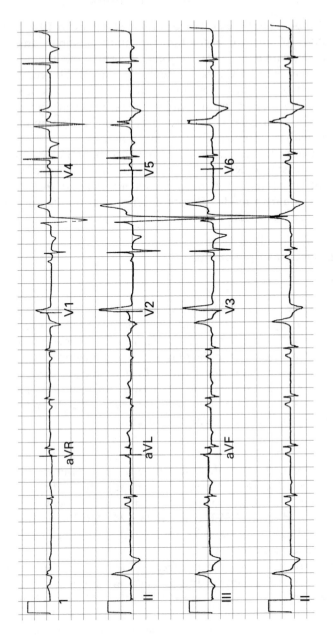

Figure 13.1 Electrocardiogram of a 19-year-old man with right ventricular dysplasia, demonstrating widespread T wave inversion and ventricular ectopic beats with a left bundle branch block morphology. He had presented with a history of palpitations induced by playing soccer: clinical examination was normal. (*From* Aziz S, McMahon RFT, Garratt CJ. Sudden cardiac death in arrhythmogenic right ventricular dysplasia. *Circulation* 2000;**101**:825–7.)

Patients are thought to have evidence of familial disease in 50% of cases. Systematic study of affected asymptomatic family members frequently reveals individuals with a milder or "concealed" form of the disease. Rarely these patients may have ECGs that are entirely normal. The condition is not known in newborns and is very rare in the first few years of life, but commonly becomes evident during adolescence. In later life presentation may be with right ventricular failure and tricuspid regurgitation or biventricular failure with requirement for transplantation.

The prevalence of the condition is estimated to be 0.6 cases for every 1000 people (at least in Italy). The 10-year cumulative survival of the condition, available in three studies only, is thought to range from 75% to 95%. The most common mode of death is ventricular fibrillation (Figure 13.2). Clinical features predictive of sudden death are:

- Family history of sudden death
- History of syncope or presyncope.

Anatomy

The characteristic features of the condition are diffuse or segmental transmural loss of the myocardium in the right ventricular free wall and its replacement by fatty or fibro-fatty tissue. There may be aneurysms of the right ventricular free wall, either due to true external bulging or "ex vacuo" hollowing at the inflow (sub-tricuspid), outflow, or apex of the right ventricle. Histology indicates some involvement of the left ventricle in approximately 50% of cases. There is often evidence of acute patchy myocarditis with myocyte necrosis and inflammatory infiltrates.

Genetics

The most common pattern of inheritance is autosomal dominant, although an autosomal recessive pattern has also been described. The remainder appear to be sporadic. Linkage analysis has defined three loci for the dominant form of the disease: ARVD1 at 14q23-q24, ARVD2 at 1q42, and ARVD3 at 14q12-q22. Some families are not linked to these loci, suggesting further genetic heterogeneity.

Despite the identification of a number of loci for the condition, the involved genes are still unknown. Interestingly, actinin genes map to the same locus as ARVD1 and 2, and segments of the actinin molecule show high homology with parts of the dystrophin molecule. Indeed, some histological features of ARVD are similar to those of muscular dystrophy and it has been suggested that the condition may be due to mutations in molecules that play in myocardial cells a similar role to the dystrophin-like protein complex.

Diagnostic criteria

The literature pertaining to this disease has suffered from the lack of uniformity of diagnostic criteria. Although this has not posed a problem in

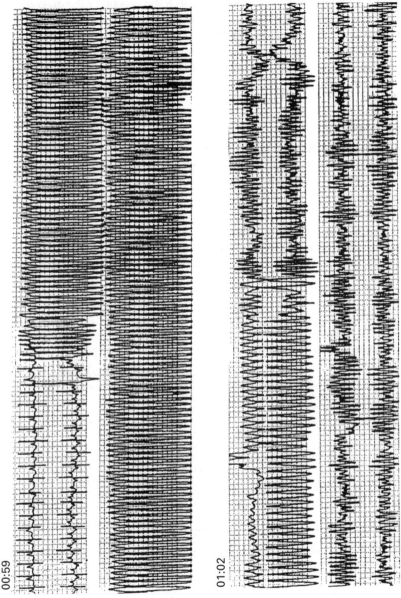

00:59

01:02

Figure 13.2   Holter recording during sudden cardiac death in the same patient as in Figure 13.1. Monomorphic VT is triggered by ventricular premature beats at 00:59 and degenerates to VF three minutes later. He was found dead outside his front door later that morning. (*From* Aziz S, McMahon RFT, Garratt CJ. Sudden cardiac death in arrhythmogenic right ventricular dysplasia. *Circulation* 2000;**101**:825–7.)

patients who have typical features, it is difficult to be certain of the diagnosis in the milder forms of the disease. Standardised criteria have now been proposed based on the presence of major and minor criteria encompassing structural, histological, electrocardiographic, and genetic factors.

The diagnosis is fulfilled by the presence of two major criteria, one major criteria plus two minor criteria, or four minor criteria from different groups (Table 13.1).

Echocardiography

A broad variety of echocardiographic abnormalities have been described. Diffuse dilatation of the right ventricle, localised bulging or aneurysms, regional akinesia, and a thickened moderator band may be present.

Angiography

Structural changes seen on echocardiography (aneurysms, areas of akinesis) can also be identified by angiography. The "pile of plates" sign (deep horizontal fissures along the anterior free wall of the right ventricle)

Table 13.1   Diagnostic criteria for right ventricular dysplasia.

1. Global and/or regional dysfunction and structural alterations[a]
   - Major
     Severe dilatation and reduction of right ventricular ejection fraction with no (or only mild) LV impairment
     Localised right ventricular aneurysms (akinetic or dyskinetic areas with diastolic bulging)
     Severe segmental dilatation of the right ventricle
   - Minor
     Mild global right ventricular dilatation and/or ejection fraction reduction with normal LV
     Mild segmental dilatation of the right ventricle
     Regional right ventricular hypokinesia
2. Tissue characterisation of walls
   - Major
     Fibro-fatty replacement of myocardium on endomyocardial biopsy
3. Repolarisation abnormalities
   - Minor
     Inverted T waves in right precordial leads (V_2 and V_3) (people aged >12 years, in absence of right bundle branch block)
4. Depolarisation/conduction abnormalities
   - Major
     Epsilon waves or localised prolongation (>110 ms) of the QRS complex in right precordial leads (V_1-V_3)
   - Minor
     Late potentials (signal-averaged ECG)
5. Arrhythmias
   - Minor
     Left bundle branch block type ventricular tachycardia (sustained and nonsustained) ECG, Holter, exercise testing).
     Frequent ventricular extrasystoles (>1000/24 h) (Holter)
6. Family history
   - Major
     Familial disease confirmed at necropsy or surgery
   - Minor
     Familial history of premature sudden death (<35 years) due to suspected right ventricular dysplasia
     Familial history (clinical diagnosis based on present criteria)

[a]Detected by echocardiography, angiography, magnetic resonance imaging, or radionuclide scitigraphy. ECG=electrocardiogram, LV=left ventricle.
Source: McKenna WJ, Thiene G, Nava A. Diagnosis of arrhythmogenic right ventricular dysplasia/cardiomyopathy. Br Heart J 1994;71:215–18.

has been said to be classical but does in fact occur in 30% of normal individuals.

Signal averaged ECG

The signal averaged ECG shows abnormalities in all of those who are obviously affected with the condition, but only 70% of those with the "concealed" forms.

Magnetic resonance imaging

Magnetic resonance imaging allows fat (high intensity, bright signal) and fibrous tissue (low intensity, dark signal) to be differentiated from normal myocardium (intermediate intensity, grey signal). In normals, adipose tissue is present in the atrioventricular groove and in the anteroapical portion of the right ventricle. Intramural or transmural fat infiltration of the right ventricular free wall is characteristic of ARVD. However, evaluation may be difficult in areas where the right ventricular wall is thin and adjacent epicardial fat is present. This is particularly true of the apex and tricuspid area of the right ventricle.

Endomyocardial biopsy

This technique may be diagnostic but is limited by sampling error, particularly as the septum, the safest place for biopsy, is usually spared.

None of the above techniques is 100% sensitive or specific for the condition and as a consequence the diagnosis relies on a combination of clinical and other features as outlined in Table 13.1. In terms of the investigation of asymptomatic family members, the disease can effectively be excluded in the presence of a completely normal ECG and echocardiogram (as long as the latter is undertaken by an experienced operator with particular attention being paid to the right ventricular views). If there is doubt, magnetic resonance imaging is probably the most appropriate next investigation. As the "checklist" approach to diagnosis suggests (Table 13.1), there is no gold standard diagnostic test for this condition.

Characteristics and mechanisms of ventricular arrhythmias

The ventricular arrhythmias associated with ARVD are always of left bundle branch block morphology. In patients with the classical form with widespread right ventricular involvement, the site of origin is often the inferior wall (with a leftward axis), whereas those with an inferior axis tend to have a more localised right ventricular outflow site. Ventricular tachycardia is inducible in about 85–90% of cases in which a spontaneous arrhythmia has been documented. These tachycardias show many of the features of a re-entrant form of arrhythmia, very similar to ventricular tachycardia associated with previous myocardial infarction.

109

The ventricular arrhythmogenicity of the disease is reasonably explained by the histopathological arrangement of surviving right ventricular myocardial cells embedded in the replacing fibro-fatty tissue. This would act as a substrate for inhomogeneous and slow conduction in the ventricle. Both the epsilon waves and late potentials on signal average electrocardiography reflect this intraventricular conduction defect.

One of the striking features of this form of ventricular tachycardia (and the one that clearly differentiates it from that associated with previous myocardial infarction) is the exercise-dependent nature of the arrhythmia. A recent study by MIBG-scintigraphy in AVRD suggested functional and/or structural sympathetic denervation in regions of left ventricular myocardium adjacent to the diseased right ventricular musculature. Since sympathetic nerve trunks travel in the subepicardium they may be damaged in AVRD, which typically progresses from the epicardium to the endocardium. Consequently, it has been proposed that denervation supersensitivity to catecholamines may explain the effort-related nature of the arrhythmias. Other suggestions include exertionally related stretch of the right ventricle as a precipitating factor.

Therapy

Patients should be told about the relationship between exercise and arrhythmias in ARVD and that vigorous sporting activities should be avoided.

Therapy in patients with ARVD is aimed at either suppressing the ventricular arrhythmias or improving cardiac function in the presence of right ventricular or biventricular failure.

There are no controlled data on treatment aimed at suppressing ventricular arrhythmias in this condition, primarily because of the relative rarity of the disease. Medical antiarrhythmic therapy is said to be effective in the majority of patients, with beta blockade (because of the exercise-related nature of the arrhythmias) and amiodarone being the most commonly used forms of therapy. Catheter ablation techniques are useful in abolishing re-entrant ventricular tachycardia with about much the same acute success as tachycardias associated with a previous myocardial infarction (70% in selected cases), although there is some evidence to suggest that this does not prevent subsequent development of ventricular fibrillation and sudden cardiac death.

A number of surgical procedures have been developed for this condition, including cryosurgery of culprit areas (mapped at the time of surgery) and also complete separation of the right ventricle from the rest of the heart (right ventricular dysarticulation).

The essential problem with determining therapy in patients with ARVD is the difficulty in predicting who will develop sudden cardiac death. There are no data on the predictive power of any diagnostic tests in this situation and indeed there is a strong clinical impression that sudden cardiac death may occur despite the absence of inducible ventricular arrhythmias or severe right ventricular disease. For this reason, many cardiologists recommend insertion of an implantable defibrillator in patients thought to be at high risk on clinical criteria, i.e. have a malignant family history, have a history of syncope or presyncope on exertion, and those young adults who insist on continuing athletic activity. The defibrillator is of course useful in these patients for management of their ventricular tachycardia using the anti-tachycardia modes of treatment, in addition to the presumed prognostic benefits.

Further reading

Marcus F, Fontaine G, Guiraudon G, *et al.* Right ventricular dysplasia: a report of 24 adult cases. *Circulation* 1982;**65**:384–98.

McKenna WJ, Thiene G, Nava A, *et al* on behalf of the Task Force of the Working Group on Myocardial and Pericardial Disease of the European Society of Cardiology. Diagnosis of arrhythmogenic right ventricular dysplasia/cardiomyopathy. *Br Heart J* 1994;**71**:215–18.

Thiene G, Nava A, Corrado D, Rossi L, Pennelli N. Right ventricular cardiomyopathy and sudden death in young people. *N Engl J Med* 1988;**318**:129–33.

Wichter T, Borggreffe M, Haverkamp W, Chen X, Breithardt G. Efficacy of antiarrhythmic drugs in patients with arrhythmogenic right ventricular disease: results in patients with inducible and non-inducible ventricular tachycardia. *Circulation* 1992;**86**:29–37.

PART III
DIAGNOSIS AND MANAGEMENT

14: Clinical management of the patient presenting with palpitation

Patients presenting with the symptom of palpitation form a large proportion of referrals to departments of cardiology and of internal medicine. In the great majority of cases the correct diagnosis can be determined at the initial consultation after careful analysis of the history, findings at clinical examination, and 12-lead ECG.

History

In the first instance it is important that the patient is allowed to tell his or her own story regarding their symptoms and other facts that they may consider relevant. It is equally important, however, to determine at an early stage the exact nature of the main symptom: different patients mean different things when they talk about "palpitations". It is very useful to ask the patient to *beat out the heart rhythm* of which they are complaining on the desk in front of you. He or she may find this difficult and prefer to describe the symptoms verbally, but they should be encouraged to persevere. At this stage it may become obvious that the patient is experiencing abnormal perception of a normal cardiac rhythm, i.e. they tap out a regular rhythm at a normal rate. Perhaps more commonly he/she will tap out a rhythm indicative of an extra beat or a "missed" beat that may indicate the occurrence of extrasystoles (the missed beat indicating a compensatory pause). Patients with symptomatic junctional tachycardias will clearly beat out a rapid regular rhythm whereas those with AF will usually indicate the irregularity of the rhythm.

The patient should be encouraged to describe in detail the approximate *number of events* that have occurred and the sequence of these events. Enquiries should be made about childhood specifically, as a very long history of palpitation indicates a congenital origin and high likelihood of junctional tachycardia. A previous history of cardiac disease and/or cardiac surgery is particularly relevant to a likely diagnosis of atrial or ventricular arrhythmias. *A history of previous myocardial infarction is strongly suggestive of a ventricular origin of palpitations.* Atrial arrhythmias may also occur in such a setting but junctional tachycardias would be unlikely.

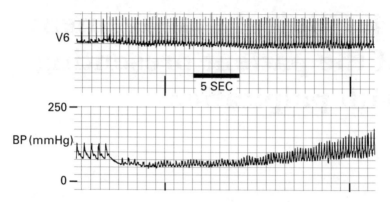

Figure 14.1 Changes in arterial blood pressure following onset of supra-ventricular tachycardia. (*From* Waxman *et al.* Reflex mechanisms responsible for early spontaneous termination of paroxysmal supraventricular tachycardia. *Am J Cardiol* 1982;**49**:259–72.)

The presence of symptoms suggestive of haemodynamic instability during tachycardia should be sought specifically. A history of *loss of consciousness* (or near loss of consciousness) in association with structural heart disease or previous myocardial infarction is strongly suggestive of a life-threatening ventricular arrhythmia. Such patients should undergo further investigation and treatment as a matter of priority. Patients with junctional tachycardia may suffer a dramatic transient fall in blood pressure and loss of conscious-ness before sympathetic activation restores it to normal or near-normal levels (Figure 14.1).

A history of *heavy alcohol intake* is relevant to the likely arrhythmia. Episodes of AF may be precipitated by "binges" of heavy alcohol intake. A long history of sustained heavy alcohol intake signals the possibility of arrhythmias associated with an alcoholic cardiomyopathy.

Patients already on antiarrhythmic therapy may develop new symptoms suggestive of the development of a new arrhythmia due to a proarrhythmic effect of a particular drug: a full *drug history* should be established. A *family history* of similar or related symptoms is clearly important in the identifica-tion of a familial condition.

Physical examination

If the arrhythmia is occurring at the time of the consultation it may be possible to go a long way towards the arrhythmia diagnosis on the basis of the examination. An irregular rhythm suggests AF or ectopy (atrial or ventricular) and a regular tachycardia suggests atrial, junctional, or ventric-ular tachycardia. Intermittent "cannon" waves in the jugular venous pulse during tachycardia indicate *atrioventricular dissociation*, usually associated with ventricular tachycardia (Figure 14.2).

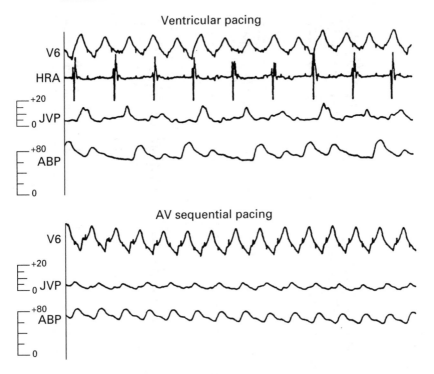

Figure 14.2 Jugular venous wave form (JVP) in simulated ventricular and supraventricular tachycardia in the same patient. (*From* Garratt CJ, Griffith MJ, Young G *et al*. Value of physical signs in the diagnosis of ventricular tachycardia. *Circulation* 1994;**90**:3103–7.)

More frequently, the principal value of the physical examination is to determine the *presence of structural heart disease* (valvular abnormalities or evidence of ventricular dysfunction) associated with the arrhythmia. This is of particular relevance to the arrhythmia diagnosis, as indicated above.

Initial diagnostic tests

The *12-lead electrocardiogram* is, of course, of great value in the diagnosis of ongoing tachycardia and this is discussed in detail in the following chapter. In addition, during sinus rhythm it can provide important circumstantial information regarding arrhythmia type. For instance, the presence of a completely normal electrocardiogram effectively excludes a diagnosis of arrhythmias associated with hypertrophic cardiomyopathy. Similarly, features suggestive of previous myocardial infarction on the electrocardiogram would suggest ventricular tachycardia as a likely arrhythmia diagnosis.

The *transthoracic echocardiogram* has a crucial role in identifying or excluding structural heart disease which, as discussed above, is very important in terms of arrhythmia diagnosis.

117

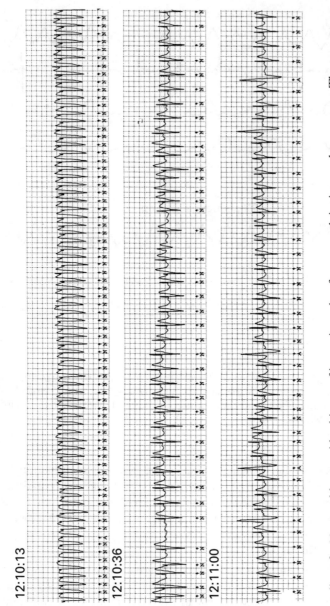

12:10:13

12:10:36

12:11:00

Figure 14.3   Holter recording of a 30 year old man with a history of intermittent but frequent palpitations and presyncope. The uppermost trace reveals a broad complex tachycardia at approximately 200 beats per minute, which changes to a narrow complex regular tachycardia at half this rate. Close examination of the second trace reveals flutter waves and subsequent electrophysiology study confirmed the presence of inducible atrial flutter.

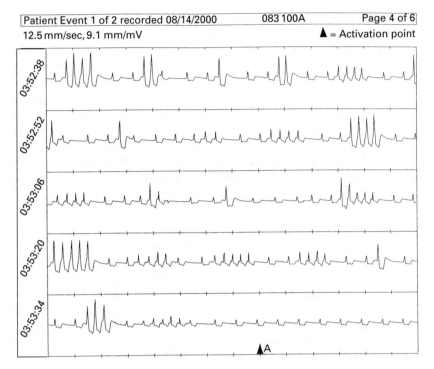

Figure 14.4 Printout from a loop recorder implanted in a 45 year old woman with infrequent palpitations. The recording shows multiple runs of narrow and wide complex tachycardia. Subsequent electrophysiology study revealed focal left atrial tachycardia.

Thyroid function tests are necessary to exclude thyrotoxicosis in cases of AF or sinus tachycardia.

Further diagnostic tests

If the patient is not in tachycardia at the time of consultation (which is the case more often than not), then further attempts may be made to record a cardiac rhythm during symptoms. This is not always necessary; for instance a patient with symptoms suggestive of intermittent atrial or ventricular ectopy in the setting of a structurally normal heart can usually be reassured without further investigation. If palpitations are occurring on a daily or near-daily basis then *ambulatory electrocardiography* (Holter monitoring) is to be recommended (Figure 14.3). The normal period of monitoring is 24 hours as the pick-up rate falls off dramatically after this period and very prolonged monitoring is impractical using this technique. If symptoms occur at a rate of one a week or less it is unlikely that Holter monitoring will be helpful and alternative methods of rhythm documentation are required. One of the most useful is the *cardiomemo*: this device can be carried in the pocket and can record cardiac rhythm during symptoms when

119

positioned by the patient on their own chest. This recorded rhythm can then be transmitted to a central monitoring station using a conventional telephone. For very intermittent symptoms, particularly if there is loss of consciousness (and consequent inability to use a handheld device), an *implantable loop recorder* is of great value. This small device (approximately $4 \times 1 \times 0.5$ cm) is implanted subcutaneously in the prepectoral region under local anaesthetic in a similar manner to a pacemaker. It monitors cardiac rhythm continuously and records episodes of tachycardia or brady-cardia both automatically and if activated by the patient at the time of symptoms (Figure 14.4). Tracings can be retrieved by telemetry and the battery life of the device is approximately 18 months. After this period (or when the diagnosis has been made) the device is explanted.

Electrophysiology study

It is very unusual for an *invasive electrophysiology study* to be required to diagnose the cause of palpitations. The usual aim of this procedure is to establish the site of origin of a previously documented tachycardia as a prel-ude to a curative catheter ablation procedure (see Chapter 17). It can be helpful, however, in excluding pathological tachycardia when symptoms are very troublesome and are causing repeated consultations and/or hospital admissions. In this situation the focus of the study is attempts at induction of tachycardia with atrial and ventricular extrastimuli.

Further reading

Garratt CJ, Griffith MJ, Young G, *et al.* Value of physical signs in the diagnosis of ventricular tachycardia. *Circulation* 1994;**90**:3103–7.

15: Diagnosis and management of acute episodes of tachycardia

This chapter discusses the diagnosis and treatment of acute arrhythmias, usually in the emergency room or coronary care unit setting.

Introduction

A 12-lead electrocardiogram is a simple non-invasive investigation that can, if correctly interpreted, provide valuable information concerning tachycardia mechanism and response to therapy. Unless the patient is sufficiently haemodynamically compromised, unconscious or about to be unconscious, a full 12-lead electrocardiogram should always be recorded. Although the ECG is of major importance in the diagnosis, the history from the patient may be equally important and should not be neglected. In particular, information about previous cardiac conditions (for example, myocardial infarction) is extremely valuable.

Classification of tachycardia ·

At the outset it is important to determine whether the tachycardia is regular or irregular, and whether the QRS complexes are narrow (less than 0.12 sec in any lead) or broad (greater than 0.12 sec).

Narrow complex regular tachycardia

The differential diagnosis of narrow complex regular tachycardia is listed below:
- Sinus tachycardia
- Atrial tachycardia
- Atrial flutter
- Atrioventricular re-entrant tachycardia
- Atrioventricular nodal re-entrant tachycardia.

Sinus tachycardia can be distinguished from other tachycardias by the normal P wave morphology and the demonstration of gradual acceleration and deceleration at the onset and offset of tachycardia (Figure 15.1). *Atrial*

121

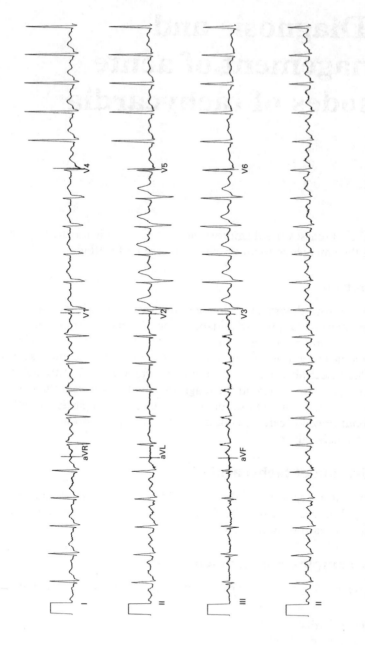

Figure 15.1   12-lead ECG of sinus tachycardia. Normal P waves can clearly be seen preceding the QRS complexes.

tachycardias are also characterised by distinct P waves preceding each QRS complex, P wave morphology being abnormal and determined by the site of origin of the tachycardia. Atrial tachycardias, unlike physiological sinus tachycardia (when AV nodal conduction may be enhanced), frequently show AV nodal Wenkebach or higher degrees of block (Figure 15.2). Regular atrial activation of approximately 300 beats/min strongly implies a diagnosis of *atrial flutter* which is frequently conducted for ventricles with 2 : 1 block resulting in a regular ventricular rate of 150 beats/min. The classic "saw-tooth" or "picket fence" appearances of the baseline between the QRS complexes characterise the typical form of atrial flutter, the flutter waves being predominantly negative in leads 2, 3, and AVF (Figure 15.3).

The position of P waves relative to the QRS complex during narrow complex regular tachycardia can give good clues to the diagnosis of *junctional tachycardias* (Figure 15.4). In patients with AV nodal re-entrant tachycardia, the small size of the re-entrant circuit and rapidity of conduction through the AV node in the retrograde direction cause the P wave to be almost synchronous with the QRS complex and therefore hidden within this complex of the surface ECG. The P waves may occasionally be identified as negative deflections within with QRS complex in the inferior leads, or as an upright deflection immediately following the RS in V1 (pseudo R wave).

Patients with orthodromic AV re-entrant tachycardia have retrograde P waves that are usually more identifiable between each QRS complex, as retrograde atrial activation follows some time after ventricular activation. These P waves may sometimes be seen as notches at the peak or at the end of the preceding T wave.

A practical approach to diagnosis and therapy of narrow complex regular tachycardia

In general three steps are involved:

1 *Identification* of P wave morphology and timing (see above).
2 *Determination of the AV relationship* during tachycardia. The presence of AV block during tachycardia excludes AV re-entrant tachycardia and strongly suggests the presence of an atrial tachycardia (Figure 15.2). Very rarely AV nodal re-entrant tachycardia may continue in the presence of AV block, the site of block being distal to the lower common pathway of the re-entrant circuit.
3 *Induction of AV block* by vagal manoeuvres and or adenosine. The Valsalva manoeuvre performed whilst the patient is lying flat is the most effective form of vagal manoeuvre in terms of production of AV block. If this fails, intravenous adenosine, as increasing bolus doses given via a peripheral vein (3 mg then 6 mg then 12 mg), is safe and has a high likelihood of succeeding in blocking AV nodal conduction for a brief period. As a consequence, junctional tachycardias will be terminated and atrial tachycardias and atrial flutter will be revealed by the transient

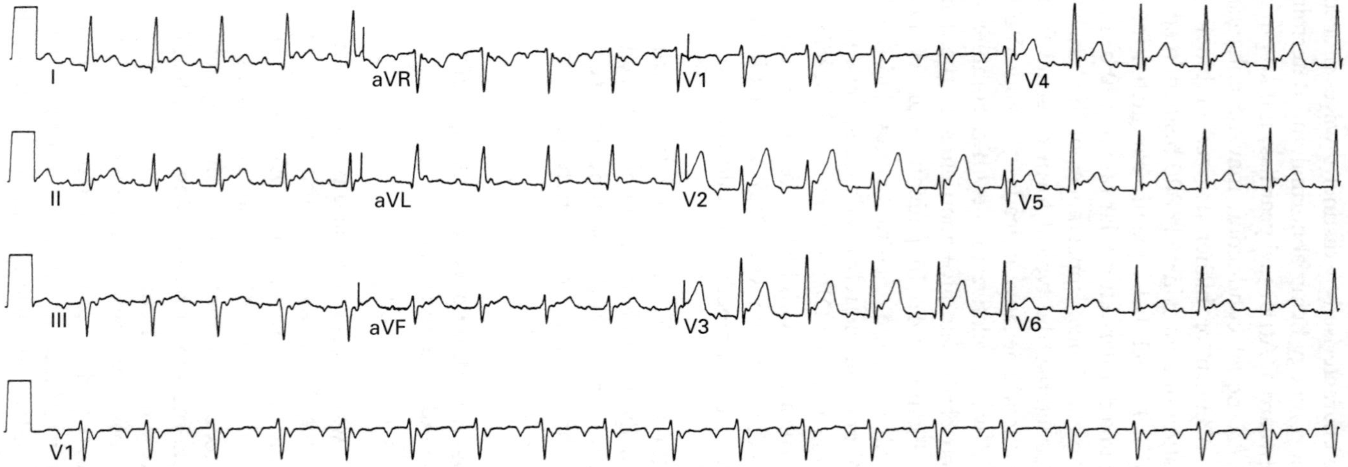

Figure 15.2 12-lead ECG of atrial tachycardia with 2:1 AV block. Distinct P waves of abnormal morphology can be seen occurring at twice the rate of the ventricular response.

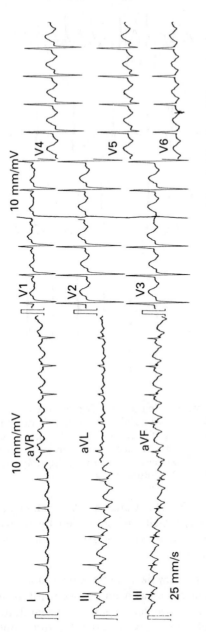

Figure 15.3   12-lead ECG of typical atrial flutter with 2 : 1 block: the characteristic negative "sawtooth" or "picket fence" flutter waves are seen in the inferior leads.

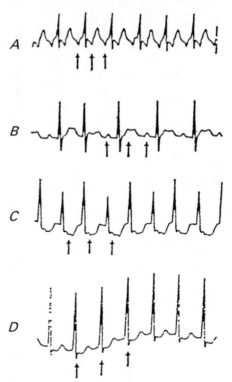

Figure 15.4   Use of P wave timing to identify the cause of narrow complex regular tachycardia. *A*: atrial flutter; *B*: atrial tachycardia; *C*: atrioventricular re-entrant tachycardia using an accessory pathway; *D*: atrioventricular nodal re-entrant tachycardia (AVNRT). All recordings are taken from standard lead II, which is usually the best for this purpose. (*From* Garratt CJ, Griffith MJ. *Electrocardiographic diagnosis of tachycardias*. Armonk, NY: Futura, 1994.)

AV block (Figure 15.5). This transient AV block occurs 10–20 seconds after injection and is usually accompanied by transient flushing and chest tightness. Adenosine may exacerbate bronchospasm and is contraindicated in asthmatics.

Intravenous verapamil is very likely to terminate junctional tachycardias in the rare case where adenosine has been unsuccessful. It may also be useful in terms of slowing the ventricular response to atrial flutter or atrial tachycardia, although this effect will last for 60–90 minutes only.

DC cardioversion is an effective therapy for most narrow complex re-entrant tachycardias. Although it is very rarely necessary in patients with junctional tachycardias, it may be used as first line treatment in patients with atrial tachycardia or atrial flutter as pharmacological therapy is often disappointing in these situations.

It should be noted that sinus tachycardia is most frequently a physiological response to anxiety, exercise, hypotension, infection, or other illness.

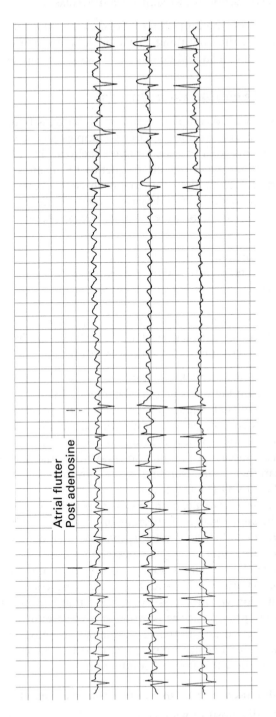

Atrial flutter
Post adenosine

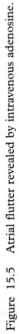

Figure 15.5   Atrial flutter revealed by intravenous adenosine.

In these situations no attempt should be made to slow the heart rate directly as it may be the only thing that is maintaining the circulation in these patients. Treatment should be directed towards the underlying cause.

Wide complex regular tachycardia

The misdiagnosis of wide complex regular tachycardia is both more common and more serious than that of narrow complex tachycardia. Patients with ventricular tachycardia or wide complex tachycardias associated with Wolff–Parkinson–White syndrome are frequently misdiagnosed as cases of SVT with aberrant conduction and inappropriately treated with intravenous verapamil, sometimes with disastrous consequences.

The differential diagnosis of wide complex regular tachycardia is listed below:

- Ventricular tachycardia
- Supraventricular tachycardia with aberrant conduction (atrial flutter, atrial tachycardia, AV re-entrant tachycardia, AV nodal re-entrant tachycardia)
- Supraventricular tachycardia with pre-excitation (atrial flutter, antidromic AV re-entrant tachycardia, AV nodal re-entrant tachycardia with a bystander activation of an accessory pathway).

Ventricular tachycardia forms the majority of cases of wide complex regular tachycardia presenting to casualty departments. They originate in ventricular myocardium itself, usually at the border of a previous myocardial infarction. For this reason, patients with wide complex tachycardia who give a history of previous myocardial infarction nearly always have ventricular tachycardia. Spread of conduction away from the site of origin is much slower than that via the Purkinje system, producing wide QRS complexes on a surface ECG (Figure 15.6).

Supraventricular tachycardia can produce a wide QRS complex under two circumstances: in the presence of aberrant or eccentric conduction to the ventricles. *Aberrant* conduction can be defined as when conduction occurs via the AV node with conduction delay occurring below this level (bundle branches or ventricular muscle). Usually it is the result of right or left bundle branch block (Figures 15.7 and 15.8). *Eccentric* conduction can be defined as conduction via an accessory pathway that bypasses the normal AV nodal route and pre-excites the ventricular myocardium. Although preexcited atrial fibrillation and flutter are the most common forms of preexcited tachycardia, certain uncommon tachycardias involving accessory pathways may also show this form of conduction.

Supraventricular tachycardia or ventricular tachycardia?

In the differential diagnosis of wide complex regular tachycardia, the most important decision is whether or not the tachycardia is ventricular in origin, as failure to diagnose VT has the worse consequences. The published

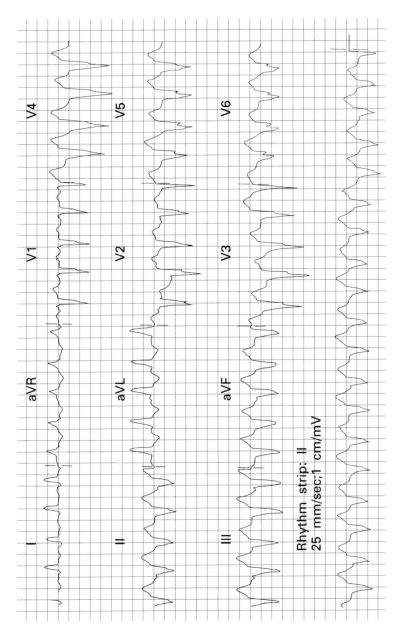

Figure 15.6 Surface electrocardiogram during ventricular tachycardia in the setting of previous myocardial infarction. QRS complexes are wide and do not have a typical left or right bundle branch block pattern.

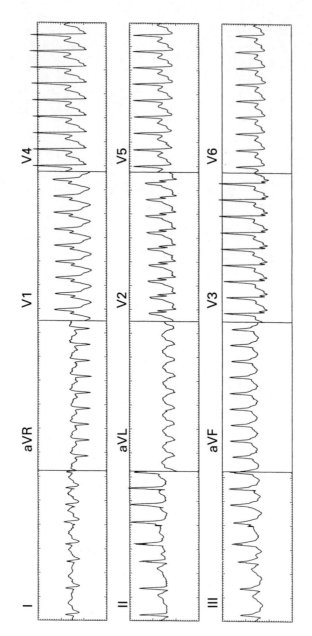

Figure 15.7 Supraventricular tachycardia with right bundle branch block.

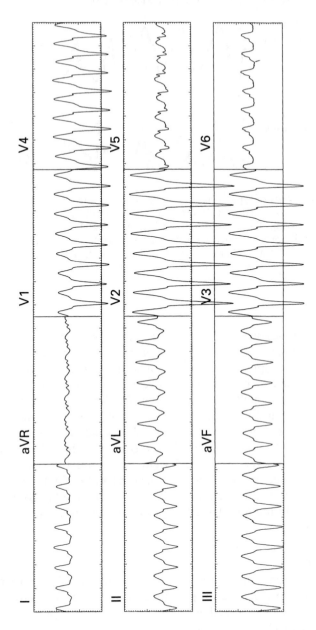

Figure 15.8   Supraventricular tachycardia with left bundle branch block.

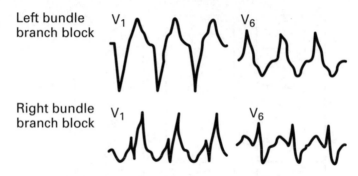

Figure 15.9   Patterns of typical right and left bundle branch block. In typical left bundle branch block pattern lead V1 shows a rapid downstroke of the S wave, with no notching or slurring. There is a dominant R wave in lead V6, with no Q wave. In typical right bundle branch block pattern there is a triphasic complex in lead V1 with the secondary R wave taller than the initial R wave. In lead V6 the R wave is taller than the S wave. (*From* Garratt CJ, Griffith MJ. *Electrocardiographic diagnosis of tachycardias*. Armonk, NY: Futura, 1994.)

electrocardiographic rules for VT diagnosis are so complex that they are not satisfied in many cases and the default diagnosis of SVT is erroneously accepted. The usual approach by inexperienced physicians is to search for independent P wave activity during tachycardia. In fact clear evidence of independent P wave activity is rarely seen in VT. A safer approach uses the reverse philosophy and attempts to make a positive diagnosis of SVT. As discussed above, aberrant conduction of SVT usually occurs as a consequence of right or left bundle branch block. Because of this, the QRS complexes are nearly always of classical right or left bundle block pattern (Figure 15.9). Recognition of these patterns identifies SVT with a high degree of sensitivity and few cases of VT are misdiagnosed as SVT. If mistakes are made (no method has 100% sensitivity and specificity), VT will be overdiagnosed.

Use of adenosine

Adenosine may assist in the diagnosis of wide complex tachycardias by terminating the majority of cases of junctional tachycardia, by producing AV block that will reveal intra-atrial arrhythmias and having no effect on VT or pre-excited atrial tachycardias (Figure 15.10). Of particular importance is the fact that adenosine is well tolerated by patients with VT, even in the presence of severe ventricular impairment.

Acute treatment of wide complex tachycardia

Adenosine is clearly of value therapeutically (in junctional tachycardia) as well as diagnostically and a suggested algorithm indicating its role is given in Figure 15.11.

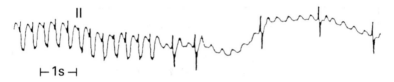

Figure 15.10 Unmasking of atrial flutter by intravenous adenosine in a 32-year-old man with dilated cardiomyopathy and a spontaneous episode of broad complex tachycardia (lead II). Fifteen seconds after the administration of 12 mg of adenosine, the ventricular rate slowed, revealing flutter waves (asterisks) occurring at a rate identical to that of the original broad complex tachycardia. (*From* Camm AJ, Garratt CJ. Adenosine and supraventricular tachycardia. *N Engl J Med* 1991;**325**:1621–9.)

Patients with VT should be DC cardioverted if there is significant haemodynamic compromise. Occasionally intravenous lidocaine may be of value in termination of well tolerated tachycardias but the success rate is not high. Intravenous amiodarone is useful, particularly if there is recurrence of tachycardia following cardioversion. Other intravenous drugs, such as disopyramide, sotalol, or flecainide, have been used with success but the efficacy rate is not high and life-threatening proarrhythmic events or worsening of ventricular function may occur. *Patients with pre-excited tachycardias* (usually patients known to have WPW syndrome, normal ventricles, with no previous history of myocardial infarction) should receive DC cardioversion if they are severely haemodynamically compromised. If the tachycardia is well tolerated then Class Ic agents such as flecainide are usually effective when given intravenously.

Irregular tachycardias (narrow or wide)

In this situation there are three main possibilities to consider.

- Atrial fibrillation with conduction to the ventricles via the AV node. This is almost certain to be the diagnosis when there is completely irregular narrow complex ventricular response with an irregular baseline and no recognisable P wave activity between the QRS complexes. If the atrial fibrillation is aberrantly conducted then the QRS complexes will have the typical left or right bundle branch shape (see Figure 15.9).
- Atrial fibrillation with pre-excitation. In this situation ventricular complexes will be broad but will not have the typical right or left bundle branch block pattern. Ventricular rate may be very high (Figure 15.12).
- Polymorphic ventricular tachycardia. Polymorphic VT is very rapid and by definition has varying QRS morphology and rate. In the setting of a long QT interval this arrhythmia is sometimes referred to as torsade de pointes, literally a "twisting of the points" (Figure 15.13). In the absence of a long QT interval in sinus rhythm, polymorphic ventricular

133

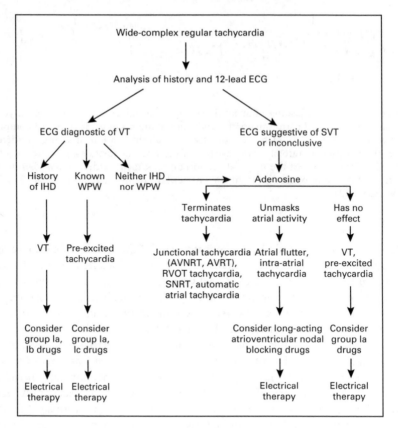

Figure 15.11   An approach to the acute management of wide complex tachycardia. (*From* Camm AJ, Garratt CJ. Adenosine and supraventricular tachycardia. *N Engl J Med* 1991;**325**:1621–9.)

tachycardia is usually associated with significant ischaemic heart disease and may be an expression of acute ischaemia or infarction.

Acute therapy of irregular tachycardias

Atrial fibrillation has a high chance of conversion to sinus rhythm with intravenous flecainide if:

- it is of short duration (less than 24 hours)
- ventricular function is normal.

This is true for pre-excited as well as non-pre-excited AF. Both digoxin and verapamil will conrol ventricular rate in non-pre-excited AF, but are likely to accelerate pre-excited AF and are contraindicated in this situation. The role of amiodarone in acute termination of AF is controversial (in that there are conflicting data about its efficacy) but it does have the advantage of

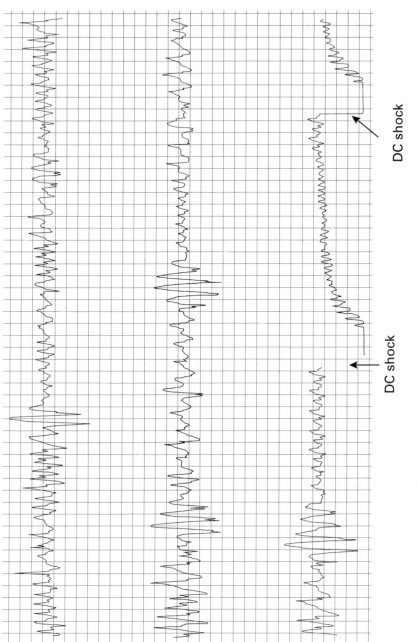

DC shock

DC shock

Figure 15.12 Pre-excited AF in a 23-year-old patient with two accessory pathways. Despite the VF-like appearance of the ECG, the patient was conscious although markedly hypotensive. An initial DC shock causes VF, only terminated by a third shock (not shown).

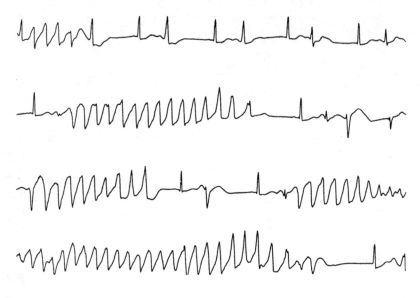

Figure 15.13 Self-terminating torsade de pointes in a patient treated with disopyramide.

being relatively unlikely to cause a proarrhythmic or hypotensive effect when used in the recommended doses.

If AF has lasted longer than 24 or 48 hours or there is likely to be left ventricular dysfunction on the basis of the previous history of cardiac disease, then pharmacological cardioversion should not be attempted as it is very unlikely to be successful. DC cardioversion should be used, using at least 200 Joules. If the arrhythmia has lasted for longer than 48 hours, formal warfarinisation will be required prior to cardioversion (see Chapter 7).

Polymorphic VT should be treated by DC cardioversion if it is sustained and with intravenous amiodarone if it is recurrent. There are few data on the role of other drugs in the acute therapy of polymorphic VT. Correction of electrolyte abnormalities and infusion of magnesium may be helpful.

Further reading

Camm AJ, Garratt CJ. Adenosine and supraventricular tachycardia. *N Engl J Med* 1991; **325**:1621–9.

Garratt CJ, Antoniou A, Ward DE, Camm AJ. Misuse of verapamil in pre-excited atrial fibrillation. *Lancet* 1989;367–9.

Garratt CJ, Griffith MJ. *Electrocardiographic diagnosis of tachycardias*. New York: Futura Publishing, 1994.

Griffith MJ, Garratt CJ, Mounsey P, Camm AJ. Ventricular tachycardia as default diagnosis in broad complex tachycardia. *Lancet* 1994;**343**:386–99.

Griffith MJ, Linker NJ, Ward DE, Camm AJ. Adenosine in the diagnosis of broad complex tachycardias. *Lancet* 1988;**1**:672–5.

Rankin AC, Rae AP, Cobbe SM. Misuse of intravenous verapamil in patients with ventricular tachycardia. *Lancet* 1987;**1**:472–4.

16: Antiarrhythmic drug therapy

How do antiarrhythmic drugs work?

It is self-evident that, given the wide variety of mechanisms of tachycardia generation, there are likely to be many different mechanisms of antiarrhythmic drug action. In Table 16.1 the proposed mechanism of action of antiarrhythmic drugs is given relative to a number of clinical arrhythmias and their proposed mechanisms. As will be appreciated from Chapters 2 and 3, some of these mechanisms (and therefore mode of action of antiarrhythmic drugs) are speculative, but the table does give a good insight into a logical approach to antiarrhythmic drug management. The part of the table that refers to "cellular" mechanisms of arrhythmia, for example automaticity and triggered activity, is the most speculative and that concerning re-entrant mechanisms the most evidence-based. As has been previously stated, re-entrant mechanisms apply to the majority of clinical arrhythmias. The approach taken in Table 16.1 (taken from the Task Force of the Working Group on Arrhythmias of the European Society of Cardiology in 1991) is that re-entrant arrhythmias with a long excitable gap are unlikely to be suppressed or terminated by increase in refractoriness. Therefore they postulate that the best approach is to depress or block conduction in the re-entrant circuit and therefore they recommend sodium-channel blocking agents. On the other hand, those arrhythmias that are thought to have a short excitable gap (including atrial fibrillation) are thought best targeted by prolonging refractoriness with potassium-channel blockers (Figure 16.1). This approach, whilst logical (and a good way to think about things in the first instance), is very much an oversimplification. The stability of the re-entrant circuit (whatever the size of the excitable gap) may be reduced or enhanced by conduction slowing or increase in refractoriness as stability of the circuit is very much dependent upon the relationship between the two. Predictions of efficacy based on assumptions about the size of the excitable gap do not hold true for all (or even most) of the time. For instance, sodium-channel blockers such as flecainide are perhaps more effective in the management of atrial fibrillation than potassium-channel blockers, and the actions of antiarrhythmic drugs are based on much more than whether they block the sodium channel (and

137

Table 16.1 Mechanisms of drug actions on arrhythmias based on modification of the vulnerable parameter.

Arrhythmia	Mechanisms	Vulnerable parameter	Drugs
	Automaticity (A) Enhanced normal		
Inappropriate sinus tachycardia		Phase 4 depolarisation (decrease)	β-adrenergic blocking agents
Some idiopathic ventricular tachycardias			Na^+-channel blocking agents
	(B) Abnormal		
Ectopic atrial tachycardia		Maximal diastolic potential (hyperpolarisation) or	M_2 agonists
		Phase 4 depolarisation (decrease)	Ca^{2+}- or Na^+-channel blocking agents
Accelerated idioventricular rhythms		Phase 4 depolarisation (decrease)	M_2 agonist Ca^{2+}- or Na^+-channel blocking agents
	Triggered activity (A) EAD		
Torsades de pointes		Action potential duration (shorten) or	β-agonists; vagolytic agents (increase rate)
		EAD (suppress)	Ca^{2+}-channel blocking agents; Mg^{++}; β-adrenergic blockers
	(B) DAD		
Digitalis-induced arrhythmias		Calcium overload (unload) or	Ca^{2+}-channel blocking agents
		DAD (suppress)	Na^+-channel blocking agents
Certain automonically mediated ventricular tachycardias		Calcium overload (unload) or	β-adrenergic blocking agents
		DAD (suppress)	Ca^{2+}-channel blocking agents, adenosine

Arrhythmia	Mechanism (target)	Drugs
Re-entry (Na$^+$-channel dependent)		
(A) Long excitable gap		
Atrial flutter type I	Conduction and excitability (depress)	Na$^+$-channel blocking agents (except lidocaine, mexiletine, tocainide)
Circus movement tachycardia in WPW syndrome	Conduction and excitability (depress)	Na$^+$-channel blocking agents (except lidocaine, mexiletine, tocainide)
Sustained monomorphic ventricular tachycardia	Conduction and excitability (depress)	Na$^+$-channel blocking agents
(B) Short excitable gap		
Atrial flutter type II	Refractory period (prolong)	K$^+$-channel blockers
Atrial fibrillation	Refractory period (prolong)	K$^+$-channel blockers
Circus movement tachycardia in WPW syndrome	Refractory period (prolong)	Amiodarone, sotalol
Polymorphic and sustained monomorphic ventricular tachycardia	Refractory period (prolong)	Quinidine, procainamide, disopyramide
Bundle branch re-entry	Refractory period (prolong)	Quinidine, procainamide, disopyramide, bretylium
Ventricular fibrillation	Refractory period (prolong)	
Re-entry (Ca^{2+}-channel dependent)		
AV nodal re-entrant tachycardia	Conduction and excitability (depress)	Ca$^+$-channel blocking agents
Circus movement tachycardia in WPW syndrome	Conduction and excitability (depress)	Ca$^+$-channel blocking agents
Verapamil-sensitive ventricular tachycardia	Conduction and excitability (depress)	Ca$^+$-channel blocking agents

Source: Task Force of the Working Group on Arrhythmias of the European Society of Cardiology: The Sicilian Gambit. A new approach to the classification of antiarrhythmic drugs based on their actions on arrhythmogenic mechanisms. *Circulation* 1991;**84**:1831–51, Copyright 1991, American Heart Association

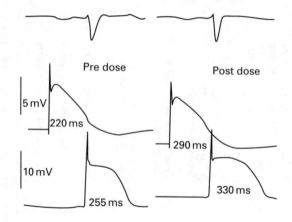

Figure 16.1   Effects of intravenous dofetilide on monophasic action potential duration in humans. There is a prolongation of both atrial and ventricular monophasic action potential durations. (*From* Cobbe S. Antiarrhythmic versus proarrhythmic effects of class III agents. In: Breithardt G, Borggrefe M, Camm J, Shenasa M, eds. *Antiarrhythmic drugs*. Berlin: Springer, 1994.)

depress conduction) or the potassium channel (and prolong refractoriness). Each individual drug has multiple actions, giving rise to a number of different classification systems of antiarrhythmic drugs (see below).

Classification of antiarrhythmic drug action

The Vaughan Williams scheme (Table 16.2)

Under this scheme antiarrhythmic drugs are classified according to which site they bind and block on the cardiac cell membrane. Thus class I drugs block the sodium channel (and slow conduction velocity), class II block adrenergic receptors (and act by blunting the effect of sympathetic stimulation on cardiac electrophysiology), class III drugs block potassium channels (and increase refractoriness), and class IV drugs block calcium channels (and slow conduction and increase refractoriness in the areas of the heart that depolarise primarily by means of calcium channels, i.e. the sinoatrial and atrioventricular nodes).

The Vaughan Williams classification further subdivides class I actions into I_A, I_B, and I_C (see Table 16.2). These differences relate to a large extent to the binding characteristics of the different drugs to the sodium channels. Although all class I drugs bind to the sodium channel, they do not bind with any permanent sense and they are constantly binding and unbinding with activation and inactivation of the channel. Drugs with actions of class I_B, for example lidocaine, unbind rapidly from the sodium channel and at normal heart rates slowing of conduction is minimal. On the other hand drugs with class I_C action unbind slowly from the channel and produce

140

Table 16.2   The Vaughan Williams classification of antiarrhythmic drugs.

Class I Drugs that delay fast sodium channel mediated conduction	Class II Sympathetic drugs	Class III Drugs that prolong repolarisation	Class IV Calcium antagonists
Ia Depress phase 0 Delay conduction Prolong repolarisation • Disopyramide • Procainamide • Quinidine	Acebutolol Betaxolol Bisoprolol Bucindolol Carvedilol Esmolol Metoprolol	Amiodarone Azimilide Bretylium Dofetilide Ibutilide Sotalol Tedisamil	Diltiazem Verapamil

Ib
Little effect on phase 0
  in normal tissue
Depress phase 0
  in abnormal tissue
Shorten repolarisation
  or little effect
• Diphenylhydantoin
• Lidocaine
• Mexiletine
• Tocainide
	Nadolol
	Propranolol
	
	Timolol
	
	Others		

Ic Markedly depress phase 0 Markedly slow conduction Slight effect on repolarisation • Flecainide • Moricizine? • Propafenone			

Source: Singh BN. Current antiarrhythmic drugs. An overview of mechanisms of action and potential clinical utility. *J Cardiovasc Electrophysiol* 1999;**10**:283–301

significant blockade at normal rates, and therefore significant conduction slowing. The success of the Vaughan Williams scheme hinges to a large extent on its ability to characterise the variable effects of class I and class III drugs on the sodium and potassium channels and on conduction velocities and refractory periods.

Site-specific classification scheme (Figure 16.2)

This form of classification, at one time referred to as the Touboul classification, simply states where a drug has its predominant site of action. Given that cardiologists think about arrhythmia mechanisms very much in terms of a site-specific system (see Chapter 4), it is not surprising that to a large extent they think about antiarrhythmic drugs in the same way. For instance, if a re-entrant tachycardia involves the AV node then it may well be susceptible to calcium-channel blocking drugs or digoxin. Alternatively,

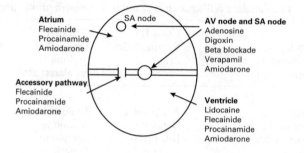

Figure 16.2   The Touboul classification of antiarrhythmic drugs, based on the primary site of action within the heart (sinus node, atrium, AV node, accessory pathway or ventricle).

lidocaine is of no use in the treatment of atrial arrhythmias and amiodarone can be used for almost any type of cardiac arrhythmia.

The Sicilian Gambit classification (Table 16.3)

This is an attempt to take into account the large number of different actions of antiarrhythmic drugs and is a much more comprehensive system which lists the actions of antiarrhythmic drugs in terms of their effects on channels, receptors, pumps, and clinical effects.

In reality, clinicians use all three systems to a greater or lesser extent and one has to be aware that the choice of an antiarrhythmic drug often reflects the relative risks of the available drugs more than (or as much as) relative efficacy. Of particular relevance in this regard is the proarrhythmic potential of antiarrhythmic drugs.

Proarrhythmic effects of antiarrhythmic drugs

Worsening of re-entrant arrhythmias by agents that slow conduction

It is apparent from the discussion in Chapter 3 that the conditions for re-entry involve a balance between conduction properties and refractoriness within any particular re-entrant circuit. To some extent the effect any particular drug will have on this balance cannot be predicted and as a consequence it is possible to make re-entrant circuits more stable rather than less so using antiarrhythmic drugs. Indeed, with the stronger conduction-slowing drugs such as flecainide, new re-entrant circuits can be formed (usually in patients with pre-existing structural heart disease) that can be life-threatening. This effect was most strikingly evident in the Cardiac Arrhythmia Suppression Trial (CAST) (Figure 16.3). As a consequence, flecainide and other class I drugs (with the exception of lidocaine) are contraindicated in patients with evidence of coronary artery disease or structural ventricular disease.

Table 16.3 The Sicilian Gambit classification of antiarrhythmic drugs.

Drug	Channels						Receptors				Pumps	Clinical effects			ECG effects		
	NA			Ca	K	I_f	α	β	M_2	P	Na-K ATPase	Left ventricular function	Sinus rate	Extra-cardiac	PR interval	QRS width	JT interval
	Fast	Med	Slow														
Lidocaine	○											↑	↑	◐			→
Mexiletine	○											↑	↑	◐			→
Tocainide	○											↑	↑	●			→
Moricizine	◐											→	↑	○			
Procainamide		Ⓐ			◐							→	↑	●	←	←	←
Disopyramide		Ⓐ			◐				○			→	↑	◐	→	←	←
Quinidine		Ⓐ			◐		○		○			↑	←→	◐	→	←	←
Propafenone		Ⓐ						◐				→	↑	○	←	←	
Flecainide			Ⓐ		○							→	↑	○	←	←	
Encainide			Ⓐ									→		○	←	←	
Bepridil	○			●	◐							?	→	○			←
Verapamil	○			●			◐					→	→	○	←		
Diltiazem				◐								→	→	○	←		

Table 16.3 Continued

Drug	Channels						Receptors				Pumps	Clinical effects			ECG effects		
	NA			Ca	K	I_f	α	β	M_2	P	Na-K ATPase	Left ventricular function	Sinus rate	Extra-cardiac	PR interval	QRS width	JT interval
	Fast	Med	Slow														
Bretylium					●		◧	◧				→	↓	○			↑
Sotalol					●			●				↓	↓	○	↑		↑
Amiodarone	○			○	◐		◐	◐				→	↓	●	↑		↑
Alinidine						●						?	↓	●	↑		
Nadolol								●				↓	↓	○	↑		
Propranolol	○							●				↓	↓	○	↑		
Atropine									●			→	↑	◐	↓		
Adenosine										□		?	↓	○	↑		
Digoxin									□		●	↑	↓	●	↑		↓

Relative potency of block: ○ Low   ◐ Moderate   ● High   A, Activated state blocker
□ Agonist   ◧ Agonist/antagonist   I, Inactivated state blocker

Source: as Table 16.1; Copyright 1991, American Heart Association

Acquired long QT syndrome

The prolongation of refractoriness by antiarrhythmic drugs has one major potential downside, that of the induction of potentially life-threatening ventricular arrhythmias. Patients with a combination of QT prolongation secondary to antiarrhythmic or other therapy and associated ventricular arrhythmias associated with this syndrome are said to have the acquired long QT syndrome. The ventricular arrhythmias are usually either self-terminating polymorphic ventricular tachycardia or ventricular fibrillation. The typical torsade de pointes characteristics of the congenital syndrome may or may not be present. There is a long list of drugs and conditions that can cause this syndrome and it is a significant consideration when prescribing antiarrhythmic drugs with class III actions (Table 16.4). The principal exception to this is amiodarone, which, despite its long list of adverse effects, has a relatively low incidence of proarrhythmic effects. Treatment of ventricular arrhythmias occurring as a result of antiarrhythmic medication is based on the following:

- Cessation of the offending drug
- Correction of electrolyte abnormalities (hypokalaemia exacerbates the acquired long QT syndrome)
- Maintenance of a relatively high heart rate by pacing (QT duration is rate-dependent, QT interval increasing with slower heart rates)
- Infusion of intravenous magnesium.

Negative inotropic effects

Nearly all antiarrhythmic drugs have negatively inotropic effects. The only exception to this is digoxin. Amiodarone has only a minor negatively inotropic

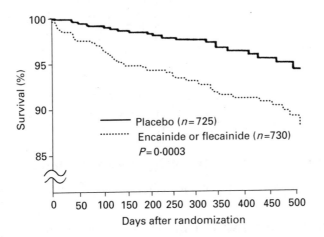

Figure 16.3 Improved survival with placebo compared with patients taking encainide or flecainide in the Cardiac Arrhythmia Suppression Trial. (*From* the CAST Investigators. Preliminary report: effect of encainide and flecainide on mortality in a randomized trial of arrhythmia suppression after myocardial infarction. *N Engl J Med* 1989;**321**:406–12.)

145

Table 16.4   Drugs known to cause acquired long QT syndrome.

Drug class	Drug (trade name)
Class IA antiarrhythmic agents	Quinidine, procainamide (Procan, Procanbid, Pronestyl), disopyramide (Norpace)
Class IC antiarrhythmic agents	Flecainide (Tambocor)
Class III antiarrhythmic agents	Amiodarone (Cordarone), sotalol (Betapace), ibutilide (Corvert), dofetilide (Tikosyn)
Calcium-channel antagonists	Bepridil (Vascor), nicardipine (Cardene)
Antihistamines	Astemizole (Hismanol), terfenadine (Seldane), diphenhydramine (Benadryl), clemastine (Tavist)
Antidepressants	Amitriptyline (Elavil, Endep), desipramine (Norpramin), doxepin (Sinequan, Zonalon), fluoxetine (Prozac), imipramine (Tofranil), venlafaxine (Effexor)
Antipsychotics	Chlorpromazine (Thorazine), haloperidol (Haldol), risoperidone (Risperdal), thioridazine (Mellaril)
Antimicrobials	Erythromycin, clarithromycin (Biaxin), grepafloxacin (Raxar), moxifloxacin (Avelox), sparfloxacin (Zagam), trimethoprim-sulfamethoxazole, amantidine, forscarnet (Foscavir), pentamidine (Pentacarinat, Pentam, NebuPent), fluconazole, ketoconazole, itraconazole, miconazole, halofantrine, chloroquine
Anticonvulsants	Felbamate (Felbatol), fosphenytoin (Cerebyx)
Miscellaneous agents	Cisapride (Propulsid), droperidol (Inapsine), naratriptan (Amerge), pimozide (Orap), probucol (Lorelco), indapamide (Lozol), sumatriptan (Imetrex), tacrolimus (Prograf), tamoxifen (Nolvadex), zolmitriptan (Zomig)

See website: http://www.dml.georgetown.edu/depts/pharmacology/torsades.html

effect. The possibility of negative inotropy must be borne in mind, particularly in patients who have impaired ventricular function already. Certainly combinations of antiarrhythmic drugs can be extremely dangerous in this respect.

A personal approach to antiarrhythmic drug therapy

My own approach to oral antiarrhythmic drug therapy is based on the following principles.

- If antiarrhythmic drug therapy can be avoided then this is the best option. Infrequent non-life-threatening arrhythmias may not need any antiarrhythmic treatment and in many other situations radiofrequency catheter ablation is more appropriate.
- If an antiarrhythmic drug is required as prophylactic therapy for a non-life-threatening arrhythmia, "safe" drugs (beta blockers, verapamil,

146

ANTIARRHYTHMIC DRUG THERAPY

digoxin) should be attempted in the first instance, even if the likely efficacy is relatively low.

- Just because a patient has suffered a recurrence of tachyarrhythmia whilst taking an antiarrhythmic drug, this does not necessarily constitute a failure of that drug therapy and requirement for institution of a different drug. Antiarrhythmic drugs are not a curative treatment and it must be expected that, for instance with paroxysmal atrial fibrillation, even with an effective drug, there may be occasional paroxysms. All too frequently physicians feel the need to change treatment in response to a single episode to a drug that may be less effective or more dangerous.
- If an antiarrhythmic agent has a life-threatening potential (for example sustained ventricular tachycardia), then amiodarone is probably the drug of first choice. An ICD should be considered in all such cases.

A description of the principal features of some commonly used antiarrhythmic drugs is given below. This description is far from exhaustive but reflects the drugs most used by the author. It is fair to say that the range of antiarrhythmic drugs prescribed by cardiologists is reducing rather than increasing, partly because of an increased awareness of the dangers of drug therapy and partly because of the emergence of non-pharmacological treatments.

Amiodarone

Amiodarone is the most powerful antiarrhythmic agent available for clinical use and has widespread efficacy in terms of suppressing arrhythmias of nearly all varieties. Unlike flecainide, it does not have high proarrhythmic potential and does not have severely negatively high inotropic effects. Its major problem, however, is its high incidence of adverse effects, which can occasionally be fatal. In terms of dosage, a long loading phase is required because the agent has a very large volume of distribution within the body fat. Usually 600 mg a day are given for one week, then 400 mg a day for a second week, and 200 mg a day thereafter. It has several mechanisms of action, but its major electrophysiological effect is the homogenous prolongation of the action potential, and therefore of refractoriness in all cardiac tissues. In addition to its potassium channel effects, amiodarone produces mild blockade of the sodium channel, a degree of beta blockade and calcium-channel blockade. In terms of its therapeutic use, amiodarone is of great value in suppressing arrhythmias that are resistant to other forms of medical therapy. It is the most effective drug ever developed for prophylaxis against ventricular tachycardia and ventricular fibrillation.

As mentioned previously, its use is limited primarily by its adverse effects, which are more likely to occur with long term use but can also occur with short term use. The most common adverse effects are photosensitivity, nausea and abnormalities of thyroid and liver function tests. The most serious adverse effect is lung fibrosis, which may be irreversible.

The incidence of death associated with the use of amiodarone is thought to be approximately 0.1% per year. Amiodarone interacts with warfarin such that the warfarin dose should be reduced whenever amiodarone is started. Many attempts have been made to design a drug with amiodarone-like efficacy but without adverse effects ("son of amiodarone") but no satisfactory replacement has emerged to date.

Atenolol

Atenolol is a beta blocker that is commonly used in the treatment of hypertension and angina. It is also an extremely valuable agent for the management of arrhythmias. Its usual dosage is 50 or 100 mg once daily. The antiarrhythmic action of beta blockers have been relatively neglected, probably because they have only a small electrophysiological effect in the normal heart. Phase IV depolarisation of sinus node cells are inhibited causing a slowing in heart rate and there is a slowing in conduction and prolongation in the refractory period of the AV node. There is very little effect on conduction velocity or refractoriness in normal atrial or ventricular myocardium. Atenolol can be useful in the control of ventricular rate during atrial fibrillation, and is often used in combination with digoxin. It may also be useful to some extent in the prophylaxis of paroxysmal atrial fibrillation and in re-entrant arrhythmias using the atrioventricular node. Possibly because of its anti-ischaemic effect, it is of value in prophylaxis against ventricular arrhythmias associated with ischaemic heart disease. Not surprisingly it is also useful in the management of catecholamine-related ventricular arrhythmias in the absence of structural heart disease. It is frequently effective for the suppression of symptomatic ventricular premature beats. Perhaps the main attraction of beta blocker therapy is its safety, although it can have negative inotropic actions. Beta blockers are the only class of antiarrhythmic agent shown convincingly to improve mortality following myocardial infarction and have no serious long term adverse effects. Many different types of beta blockers are in current use (for example metoprolol, nadolol) with similar efficacy and safety profiles.

Digoxin

Digoxin is one of the most frequently prescribed medications for the treatment of atrial arrhythmias. Its principal electrophysiological effect is slowing of AV node conduction and prolongation of AV node refractory period. The elimination half-life of digoxin is 20–30 hours and the usual dosage is 0.25 mg a day. Digoxin is used principally for the slowing of ventricular rate during established atrial fibrillation, although it may also be of value in re-entrant tachycardias that involve the AV node. As with verapamil, it is contraindicated in patients with the Wolff–Parkinson–White syndrome. Digoxin is a relatively safe antiarrhythmic agent, but in high concentrations (particularly likely in elderly patients with renal dysfunction) can cause atrial arrhythmias and ventricular arrhythmias with severe toxicity. Digoxin remains unique in that it is the only drug that prolongs refractoriness at the AV node whilst augmenting myocardial contraction. This is what gives it its particular value in atrial fibrillation when the ventricular function is impaired or unknown.

Flecainide

Flecainide is one of the most powerful conduction-slowing drugs available, and as a consequence can be both of great value in some circumstances and potentially dangerous in others. The usual dosage is 100 mg twice daily with a maximum dose of 200 mg twice daily, with an elimination half-life of 12–24 hours. The major electrophysiological feature of flecainide is prolongation of QRS interval at high dosage reflecting slowing of intraventricular conduction. The drug depresses conduction in all areas of the heart. It has a significant negative inotropic effect and is contraindicated in patients with impaired left ventricular function. Currently its primary use is as a prophylactic agent in the management of paroxysmal atrial fibrillation. It is thought to prevent perpetuation of atrial fibrillation by slowing conduction preferentially at sharply turning electrical wave fronts such as those occurring in atrial fibrillation (see Chapter 3). Prior to the widespread use of radiofrequency catheter ablation, flecainide was used frequently for patients with the Wolff–Parkinson–White syndrome as it causes conduction block in accessory pathways. Flecainide is also extremely successful in suppressing ventricular arrhythmias and was used frequently for this purpose until the publication of the Cardiac Arrhythmia Suppression Trial which showed that use of the agent in patients with coronary artery disease led to an increase in mortality, despite evidence of suppression of ventricular arrhythmias. This increase in mortality has been attributed to serious proarrhythmia and the agent is now considered contraindicated in patients with cardiac ischaemia or impaired left ventricular function. Propafenone is a very similar drug, with similar uses and similar problems.

Verapamil

Verapamil is the most commonly used calcium antagonist in the management of cardiac arrhythmias. The usual dosage is 240–360 mg a day in divided doses. It has a short elimination half-life (5–12 hours). Its major electrophysiological effects are limited to the sinus and AV nodes, causing depressed automaticity, slowing of conduction, and increase in refractoriness. There is minimal or no electrophysiological effect on the atrial or ventricular myocardium. The principal use of verapamil as an antiarrhythmic agent is as a means of controlling ventricular rate during atrial tachycardia, flutter, or fibrillation. Before the widespread application of catheter ablation techniques, verapamil was frequently used for prophylaxis of AV nodal re-entrant tachycardia and re-entrant tachycardias involving concealed

149

accessory pathways. Verapamil is contraindicated in patients with accessory pathways that are capable of conducting from atrium to ventricle as this agent has no conduction-blocking effect on accessory pathways and may increase the ventricular rate of pre-excited atrial fibrillation, occasionally with the development of ventricular fibrillation (principally with intravenous verapamil). Verapamil may also be a successful prophylactic treatment for some forms of idiopathic ventricular tachycardia (see Chapter 8). Its principal problems are those of bradycardia and negative inotropy, although these are much more of a problem with the intravenous form of the agent.

Further reading

The Cardiac Arrhythmias Suppression Trial (CAST) Investigators. Preliminary report of encainide and flecainide on mortality in a randomized trial of arrhythmia suppression after myocardial infarction. *N Engl J Med* 1989;**321**:406–12.

Task Force of the Working Group on Arrhythmias of the European Society of Cardiology: The Sicilian Gambit. A new approach to the classification of antiarrhythmic drugs based on their action on arrhythmogenic mechanisms. *Circulation* 1991;**84**:1831–51.

Vaughan Williams EM. Classification of antiarrhythmic drugs. In: Sandoe E, Flensted-Jensen E, Ollsen KH (eds). *Cardiac arrhythmias*. Sodertalje, Sweden: Astra, 1970.

17: Electrophysiologic studies and radiofrequency catheter ablation techniques

The primary aim of this book, as stated in the introduction, is to explain cardiac arrhythmias and their clinical management in terms of underlying mechanisms. It is not intended to be a manual of cardiac electrophysiological techniques and the reader is referred to a number of other texts (see Further Reading below) for more detailed discussion of these aspects. It is clearly important, however, that doctors looking after patients with cardiac arrhythmias should have an understanding of the aims, limitations, and complications of electrophysiologic studies and radiofrequency catheter ablation procedures.

Electrophysiologic studies

Purpose of electrophysiologic studies

The usual aim of an electrophysiologic study (EPS) is to establish the site of origin of a tachycardia as a prelude to a curative catheter ablation procedure. Consequently it is relatively unusual for an EPS to be performed purely as a stand-alone diagnostic procedure. This latter situation may occur, however, when the aim is to assess prognostic risk. Risk assessment may be an issue in patients with abnormal ventricular function presenting with rapid palpitations, wide complex tachycardia of uncertain origin, or syncope. These patients may be experiencing rapid VT and may benefit from an implantable cardioverter defibrillator.

Technique of electrophysiologic studies

The complexity of the investigation depends upon the information already obtained about the tachycardia from surface electrocardiography and other methods. In patients in whom a junctional or atrial tachycardia is suspected (narrow complex regular tachycardia) then a full study is usually recommended. This involves recording of local electrical activity from at least the right atrium, the left atrium (usually from recordings within the coronary sinus), the His bundle position and the right ventricle (Figure 17.1). In patients in whom a ventricular tachycardia is being sought, a His bundle catheter and a right ventricular catheter may be all that is required. In patients known to have a form of atrial flutter, a multielectrode catheter is

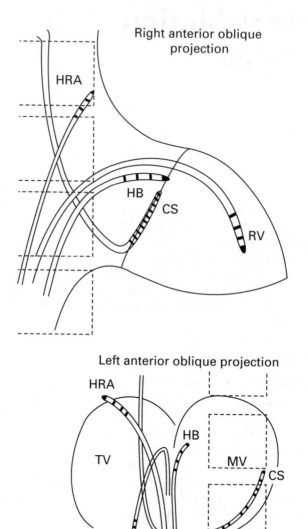

Figure 17.1   Position of electrode catheters and accompanying electrograms for a standard diagnostic electrophysiology study (orientation as for Figure 6.9) CS= coronary sinus mapping electrode, HB=His bundle electrode, HRA=high right atrial electrode, MV=mitral ring, RV=right ventricular electrode, TV=tricuspid ring.

152

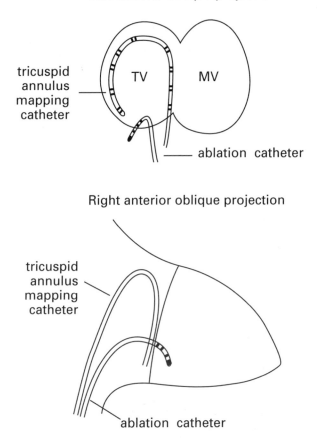

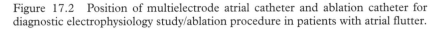

Figure 17.2 Position of multielectrode atrial catheter and ablation catheter for diagnostic electrophysiology study/ablation procedure in patients with atrial flutter.

positioned so as to record the sequence of atrial activation along the right atrial free wall and interatrial septum (Figure 17.2).

Catheters are introduced via the right femoral vein (to reach the right atrium, right ventricle, and His bundle positions) and the right internal jugular vein (for cannulation of the coronary sinus) using local anaesthetic and intravenous sedation. If detailed multielectrode mapping of the coronary sinus is not required, this structure may be cannulated from the right femoral vein.

Making a diagnosis at electrophysiologic study

The first step is usually to determine whether electrical conduction over the AV junction is normal, involves an accessory pathway, or dual AV nodal pathways. This is established by introducing premature ventricular and atrial premature beats during pacing from the right ventricle and (subsequently) the right atrium (Figures 17.3 and 17.4). Atrial stimulation

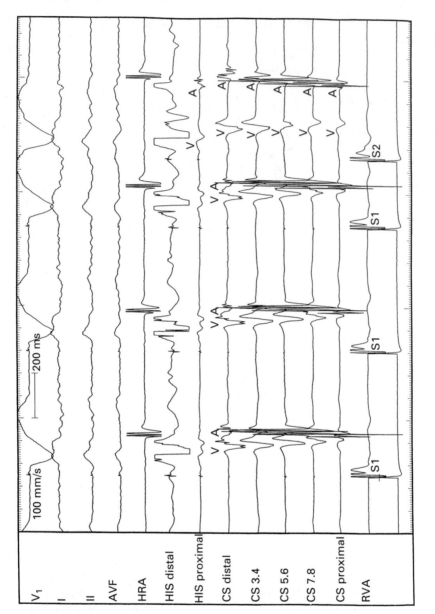

Figure 17.3 Normal ventriculo-atrial conduction pattern during ventricular pacing suggestive of conduction over the AV node. Atrial activation occurs first at the level at the proximal His bundle electrode, followed shortly after by the proximal coronary sinus (CS). A premature ventricular paced beat (S2) leads to an increase in ventrico-atrial (VA) conduction time (decremental conduction) with no change in atrial activation sequence.

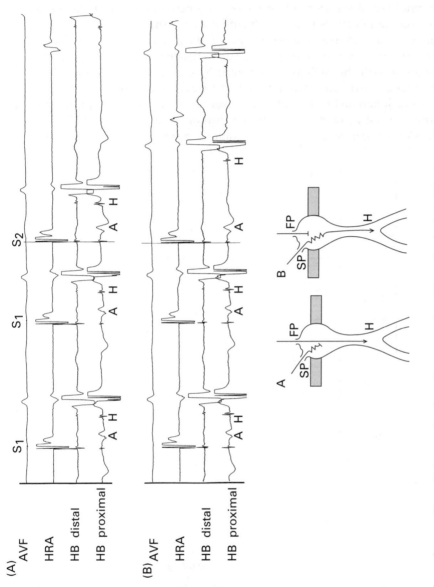

Figure 17.4 Sudden prolongation or "jump" in conduction time over the AV node (atrium–His interval) caused by increasing prematurity of an atrial extrastimulus. In panel A an atrial extrastimulus (S2) is conducted with only a small increase in AH time, suggestive of conduction over the fast AV nodal pathway. In panel B delivery of a slightly (10 ms) earlier S2 leads to block in the fast pathway and conduction over the slow AV nodal pathway, leading to a marked "jump" in AH interval.

is left until last as it may result in the development of AF which may need DC cardioversion or result in the abandonment of the study.

The second (and most important) step in diagnosis is the stimulation of tachycardia and recording of the cardiac activation sequence during the tachycardia itself. Stimulation is achieved by the introduction of atrial or ventricular extrastimuli, often during the first step of the study as described above. For junctional tachycardias the most important piece of diagnostic information is the site of earliest atrial activation during tachycardia, as this indicates the atrial insertion of the relevant accessory pathway or AV nodal

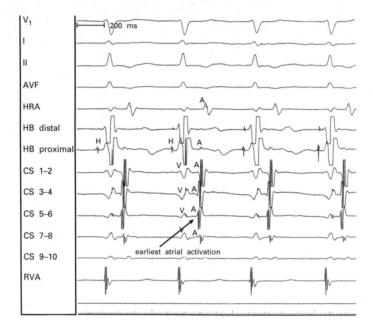

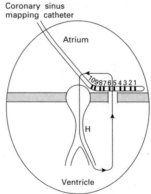

Figure 17.5   Atrial activation sequence during orthodromic tachycardia. Earliest atrial activation (*arrowed*) during tachycardia occurs at a point midway down the coronary sinus electrode, indicating a left-sided accessory pathway.

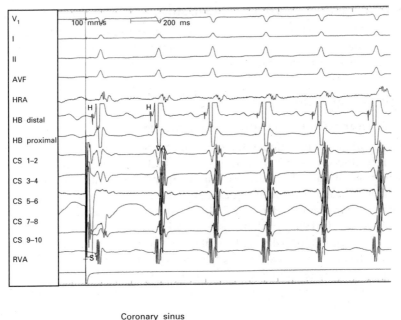

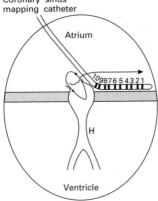

Figure 17.6   Atrial activation sequence in typical AVNRT. Atrial (A) and ventricular (V) activation are nearly simultaneous. Activation of the coronary sinus electrodes occurs in a proximal (9–10) to distal (1–2) pattern, as earliest atrial activation occurs at the fast pathway of the AV node.

pathway (Figure 17.5). In AVNRT, activation of atrium and ventricle occurs almost simultaneously, producing a characteristic "straight line" appearance of electrograms (Figure 17.6). In cases of ventricular tachycardia, atrial activity may be dissociated from ventricular activity.

As is usual with most forms of re-entrant arrhythmias, tachycardia termination can be achieved by the introduction of atrial or ventricular premature stimuli or with the use of overdrive pacing.

Complications of electrophysiologic study

This is a very low risk procedure relative to other intracardiac procedures, the principal risks being those of venous cannulation. Cardiac tamponade is possible but extremely rare in experienced hands.

Catheter ablation techniques

Brief history of catheter ablation techniques

Catheter ablation techniques for the management of cardiac arrhythmias were introduced in 1982–3, with the use of high energy DC shocks for the destruction of the AV node/His bundle in patients with AF and rapid ventricular rates. This technique required general anaesthetic and the associated barotrauma of the DC shocks caused a number of significant complications. In 1987 a radiofrequency (RF) energy source was developed for use in conjunction with deflectable electrode catheters, allowing heat-induced destruction of limited areas of myocardium around the electrode catheter tip. This technique does not require general anaesthetic and has proved to be ideal for cure of arrhythmias caused by anatomic forms of re-entry and "focal" sources.

Indications for an RF catheter ablation procedure

The specific indications for RF catheter ablation have already been discussed in relation to the individual arrhythmias but will be briefly summarised here:

- Atrial tachycardias
- Atrial flutter
- "Focal" AF
- Junctional tachycardias including those associated with the WPW syndrome
- VT in the setting of a structurally normal heart
- Bundle branch re-entrant tachycardia
- VT in the setting of previous myocardial infarction.

Ablation techniques

The essentials of ablation technique consist of (1) finding the location of the abnormal re-entrant circuit or automatic focus (see EPS above), (2) positioning the ablation catheter at a critical point in the circuit (for instance on the atrial insertion of an accessory pathway), and (3) heating up of the catheter tip using RF energy, usually for 30–60 seconds for each delivery of energy. A catheter tip temperature of 50–55 °C is usually sufficient for permanent destruction of myocardial tissue. Energy delivery may be associated with chest tightness and is usually performed under sedation and intravenous analgesia. For access to left-sided accessory pathways, left atrial or left ventricular sites, one of two approaches can be used. The

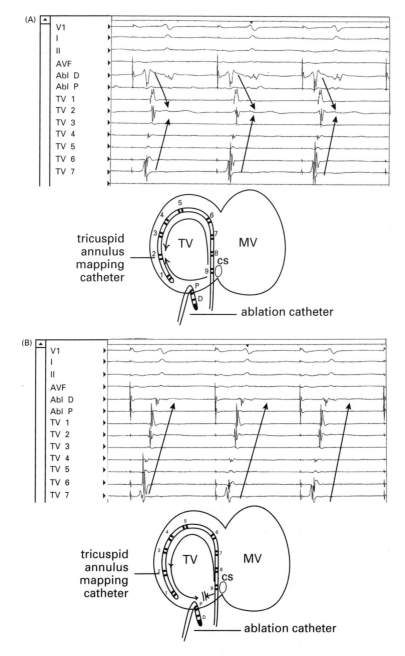

Figure 17.7 A. Pacing from the coronary sinus prior to ablation results in a "chevron" pattern of atrial activation on the tricuspid annulus electrode, as conduction to the right atrial free wall occurs via both the tricuspid isthmus and the interatrial septum. Abl D=distal electrode on ablation catheter, Abl P=proximal electrode on ablation catheter. B. Following ablation at the tricuspid isthmus the "chevron" pattern is abolished as conduction occurs via the interatrial septum only.

transaortic or retrograde approach involves insertion of the ablation catheter into the femoral artery and advancement up the aorta, across the aortic valve, and into the left ventricle (Figure 7.10). The transeptal approach involves insertion of the ablation catheter into the left atrium via a transeptal sheath.

Markers of successful ablation

In patients with the WPW syndrome successful ablation results in loss of the delta wave on the surface ECG and loss of retrograde conduction via the accessory pathway. In patients with AVNRT end points include loss of dual AV nodal physiology and inability to induce tachycardia. In patients with atrial flutter the best marker of long term success is the demonstration of bidirectional conduction block in the isthmus between the tricuspid valve and inferior vena cava (Figure 17.7).

Success rate

Acute success rate (success at the end of the procedure) approaches 95% for junctional tachycardias, atrial flutter, and idiopathic VT, although there is perhaps a 5% recurrence rate in addition, recurrence of conduction occurring within the first few days of the procedure. Success rate for atrial tachycardia and VT is currently somewhat lower than this, depending very much on case selection.

Complications of RF catheter ablation

The complications associated with RF catheter ablation are dependent upon the specific procedure being undertaken.

Slow pathway AV nodal ablation is associated with a 2% risk of complete heart block, with a lower (but still present) risk of heart block associated with midseptal or posteroseptal accessory pathways.

Ablations undertaken on the left side of the heart (left-sided accessory pathways, left atrial tachycardias, focal AF) carry a <1% risk of embolic events.

Cardiac tamponade may occur with ablation of freewall accessory pathways or with use of the transeptal puncture technique (<1%).

Coronary artery damage (and death) can (very rarely) occur with the transaortic technique for ablation of left-sided accessory pathways.

Further reading

Fogoros R. *Electrophysiologic testing*, 3rd edn. Boston, MA. Blackwell Science, 1999.
Josephson ME. *Clinical cardiac electrophysiology: techniques and interpretations.* 2nd edn. Philadelphia: Lea and Febiger, 1993.

18: Implantable cardioverter defibrillators (ICDs)

The high efficacy of direct current (DC) shock in the termination of ventricular tachycardia was demonstrated by Lown and coworkers in the 1960s, and by 1980 an implantable form of defibrillator had been described in humans. The first device to be developed was a pure cardioverter defibrillator, requiring open heart surgery for electrode patches to be placed on the heart connected to a bulky defibrillator can placed subcutaneously in the abdomen under separate incision. Second generation devices incorporated backup antibradycardia pacing, and third generation devices also incorporated the ability to terminate ventricular tachycardias with bursts of rapid ventricular pacing (Figure 18.1). In recent years these devices have become much less bulky and are implanted pre-pectorially in the same way as a bradycardia pacemaker. In general a single endocardial defibrillation electrode is implanted with a shock being delivered between this electrode and the defibrillator can (Figure 18.2).

The effect of ICDs on sudden arrhythmic death

There is little doubt that ICDs are effective in the acute termination of ventricular tachycardia and VF irrespective of the underlying cause and this has been confirmed repeatedly since Mirowski's original demonstration; few therapies offer such dramatic evidence of their efficacy (Figure 18.3). It is self-evident that reduction or abolition of sudden death by the ICD is likely to be reflected in similar effects on all cause mortality only in those patients who do not have other (non-arrhythmic) modes of death. As discussed in the previous chapter, a proportion of patients with ventricular tachyarrhythmias may well die from causes other than an arrhythmic event. As a consequence, the effect of the ICD on overall survival is critically dependent upon the sudden arrhythmic death rate in a particular patient population. The effect of the ICD on total mortality has been studied in a number of specific patient groups.

- Patients presenting with poorly tolerated ventricular tachycardia or VF outside the setting of acute myocardial infarction. Such patients were enrolled in the AVID (Antiarrhythmics versus Implantable Defibrillators) trial.

161

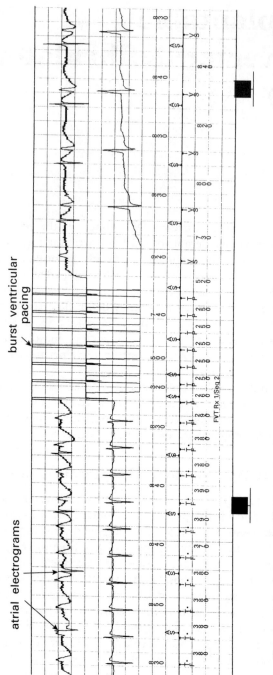

Figure 18.1 Termination of re-entrant VT by anti-tachycardia pacing from an ICD. In this case the recordings are from the endocardial leads themselves (electrograms) rather than the surface ECG. The ventricular channel is the lower of the two traces illustrated, showing VT at a rate of approximately 150 beats per minute. The upper (atrial) channel demonstrates atrial activity occurring independently at a rate of approximately 65 beats per minute. The VT is terminated by a train of seven ventricular paced beats. The numbers below the traces refer to the cycle length (number of milliseconds between two successive beats) of the tachycardia.

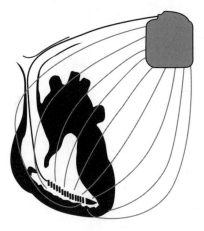

Figure 18.2   In current devices the defibrillation shock is delivered between the right ventricular electrode and the defibrillator can itself.

In this trial of just over 1000 patients, patients were randomised to implantation of an ICD or the use of antiarrhythmic drugs (primarily amiodarone or sotalol). After a mean follow-up of approximately three years there was significant survival benefit in the ICD group (Figure 18.4). Other "secondary prevention" trials such as CASH (Cardiac Arrest Study Hamburg) and CIDS (Canadian Implantable Defibrillator Study) have shown similar trends in favour of ICD therapy.

- Patients with no documented sustained ventricular arrhythmias but judged to be at high risk of arrhythmic death following myocardial infarction, i.e. with non-sustained ventricular tachycardia, impaired ventricular function, and inducible sustained ventricular arrhythmias at electrophysiology study. This group of patients were studied in the MADIT trial. This study was the first randomised study performed in patients with defibrillators and also showed significant benefit conferred by the ICD for patients with these particular selection criteria. The Multicentre UnSustained Tachycardia Trial (MUSTT) enrolled a similar group of patients in a more complicated trial design and demonstrated a similar benefit of the ICD. These trials are referred to as "primary prevention" trials as they were performed in patients who had yet to demonstrate evidence of sustained ventricular arrhythmias.

Assessment of patients prior to implantation of an ICD

History

Patients with a history of cardiac arrest or poorly tolerated ventricular tachycardia with no evidence of acute ischaemia/infarction have a high incidence of subsequent sudden death and an ICD is indicated.

163

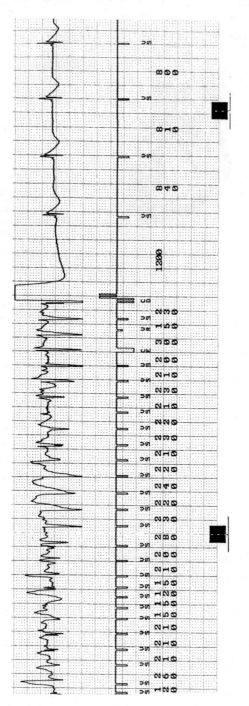
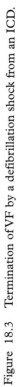

Figure 18.3   Termination of VF by a defibrillation shock from an ICD.

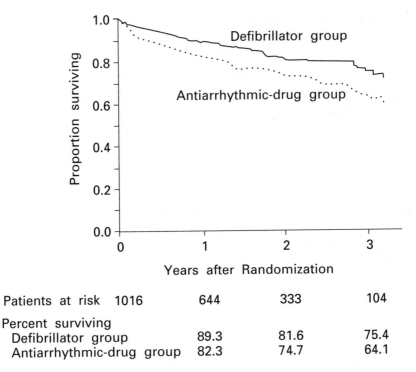

Figure 18.4 Increased survival in patients with ICDs in the AVID trial. (*From* the AVID investigators. A comparison of antiarrhythmic drug therapy with implantable defibrillators in patients resuscitated from near-fatal ventricular arrhythmias. *N Engl J Med* 1997;**337**:1576–83.)

Assessment of left ventricular function and coronary anatomy

Those patients at highest risk of arrhythmic death are those with significantly impaired left ventricular function. Patients with extremely poor left ventricular function (ejection fraction 5–10%) are likely to have a very poor prognosis irrespective of implantation of an ICD however, and many cardiologists would be reluctant to implant a device in this situation. As discussed in Chapter 9, knowledge of coronary anatomy is important in order to identify any prognostic need for revascularisation procedures.

Electrophysiologic evaluation

Patients presenting with AVID-type criteria (poorly tolerated VT or VF) do not require electrophysiologic evaluation prior to implantation of the device. Patients who are candidates for the ICD as a form of primary prevention group require it as the presence of inducible ventricular tachycardia was an important selection component of the primary prevention studies discussed above.

Indications and contraindications for implantation of the device

A number of different national and international bodies have produced guidelines for ICD implantation based upon the results of the trials discussed above. The indications are in a phase of rapid expansion but include the following.

Indications

- Resuscitated sudden death due to documented ventricular tachycardia or ventricular fibrillation in the absence of myocardial infarction within 48 hours (very good evidence).
- Sustained poorly tolerated ventricular tachycardia in the absence of myocardial infarction within 48 hours (very good evidence).
- Drug resistant recurrent haemodynamically stable ventricular tachycardia. This patient group has a relatively good prognosis and therefore it may be (although not tested) that the ICD would not confer any prognostic benefit in this group. Nevertheless, repeated hospital admissions are associated with high costs, both in financial terms and in terms of patient morbidity. In this situation, implantation of a device with both shocking and antitachycardia pacing capabilities may be a useful alternative to catheter ablation techniques.
- Patients judged to be at high risk of arrhythmic death following myocardial infarction as assessed by the presence of non-sustained VT, an ejection fraction of less than 35%, and inducible ventricular tachycardia at electrophysiologic study (very good evidence).
- ICDs may be the best option in a number of other, rarer situations, for instance in high risk patients with hypertrophic cardiomyopathy, arrhythmogenic RV dysplasia, congenital long QT syndrome, or Brugada syndrome.

Contraindications

The ICD is absolutely contraindicated in patients with very frequent sustained arrhythmias or incessant ventricular tachycardia.

Implantation of device

The development of the transvenous approach to ICD implantation represents a dramatic improvement in the role of this device and it can be performed under heavy sedation. Venous access is achieved through the subclavian vein or cephalic vein, and the defibrillation electrode with a large distal coil is passed to the right ventricular apex. This electrode is then connected to the defibrillator can in the same way as for a pacemaker and the can is buried either below the pectoral muscles or subcutaneously. At the time of implantation, the ability of the device to defibrillate appropriately is tested by the induction of ventricular defibrillation using ventricular stimulation techniques. Once satisfactory defibrillation has been demonstrated the device is programmed to deliver defibrillation shocks automatically on the recognition of ventricular tachycardia or ventricular fibrillation and, if appropriate, automatic antitachycardia pacing will also be programmed.

Complications of ICDs

The immediate complications of ICDs are those of pacemaker implantation, i.e. pneumothorax and infection. The most common complication that is specific to the device is the occurrence of inappropriate shocks, usually in response to the occurrence of atrial fibrillation. If a patient suffers frequent shocks he/she is usually admitted to hospital for interrogation of the device. If there is evidence that the shock is inappropriate then either (1) therapy directed at the atrial fibrillation can be initiated or (2) the programming of the device may be altered in order to minimise the problem.

Cost of the device

ICDs are expensive items, currently costing £16 000–20 000, and although the efficacy of the device in specific patient groups is not questioned, the average life years saved is relatively small. In AVID and CIDS, for instance, the cost per life year saved (cost-effectiveness) was £73 000 and £91 000 respectively. In terms of primary prevention, MADIT reported an average gain of 0.8 life years at a cost of £17 000 per life year, an artificially low figure that did not include substantial screening costs. Improved risk stratification is one potential future solution to the relatively modest cost-effectiveness associated with ICD treatment.

Further reading

Antiarrhythmics versus Implantable Defibrillator (AVID) Investigators. A comparison of antiarrhythmic drug therapy with implantable defibrillators in patients resuscitated from near fatal ventricular arrhythmias. *N Engl J Med* 1997;**337**:1576–83.

Moss AJ, Jackson Hall W, Cannom DS, *et al.* Improved survival with an implanted defibrillator in patients with coronary disease at high risk for ventricular arrhythmia. *N Engl J Med* 1996;**335**:1933–40.

Pathmanathan RK, Lau EW, Cooper J, *et al.* Potential impact of antiarrhythmic drugs versus implantable defibrillators on the management of ventricular arrhythmias: the Midlands trial of empirical amiodarone versus electrophysiologically guided intervention and cardioverter implant registry data. *Heart* 1998;**80**:68–70.

19: Concluding remarks

As stated in the introduction to this book, the aim has been to put forward a logical approach to arrhythmia management based on what is known about underlying mechanisms. In some instances, arrhythmias can now be explained in terms of an underlying inherited molecular abnormality, providing a great leap forward in our understanding of, for example, one form of "idiopathic" ventricular fibrillation. It is occasionally stated that "one day" all cardiac arrhythmias will be understood at a molecular level, but it is to be hoped (and indeed it is necessary) that much more than this will be achieved. The molecular bases of some clinical conditions, such as certain forms of the long QT syndrome, are known but to suggest that as a consequence we approach a full understanding of even this syndrome is to be naïve in the extreme. Genetic heterogeneity is the rule rather than the exception and for any particular form of arrhythmia substrate there are many different molecular abnormalities. For instance, prolongation of the action potential can be caused by a whole range of abnormal currents (some increased in function, some decreased), and each abnormality can be caused by a range of specific anomalous coding sequences. The smallest functional unit supporting a cardiac arrhythmia is a single cell, not a single channel, and certainly not a single amino acid substitution. The adverse effects of an inherited ion channel abnormality may be counteracted by a drug with effects on an unrelated current that results in a favourable change in action potential duration. In terms of therapy, which in the end is what we and our patients are most interested in, the unravelling of the arrhythmia substrate at cellular level is likely to be just as important as that at the molecular level.

If a single cell is the smallest functional unit supporting a cardiac arrhythmia, it is certainly not the most common. The most frequent and most dangerous form of ventricular arrhythmia is that which occurs in the setting of a previous myocardial infarction and is caused by abnormalities of propagation of electrical impulses *between* cardiac cells. Such re-entrant rhythms cannot be understood fully by the study of single myocytes and meaningful research requires an approach at the tissue level at least. Other arrhythmias, such as atrial fibrillation, may depend upon properties of the whole intact heart for their maintenance and recent advances have stemmed from the study of whole animal models.

The past few years have seen great advances in the treatment of cardiac arrhythmias, with the development of cures for AV nodal re-entrant tachycardia, accessory pathway-mediated tachycardias, idiopathic VT, the common form of atrial flutter, and certain types of atrial fibrillation. All of these advances have come directly from the study of patients in the clinical cardiac electrophysiology laboratory and owe little to more "basic" forms of research. Similarly, we may have some understanding of the way certain antiarrhythmic drugs work in single cells and in individual patients but a knowledge of their effects in large populations of patients has been shown to be vital to safe clinical practice.

Patients with arrhythmias depend upon their doctors to take a practical, individualised approach to their care based on known facts and proven treatments. Although an understanding of arrhythmia mechanisms at molecular, cellular, whole organ, and clinical levels is not always essential to good patient management, in my opinion it makes it much more likely to be achieved.

Index

Page numbers in **bold** type refer to figures; those in *italic* to tables or boxed material

accessory pathway mediated re-entrant
  tachycardia
  antidromic form 60, 62
  atrial fibrillation in 61–2, **66**, 68
  diagnosis 66, **126**
  electrophysiology studies 153–7
  mechanism **29**, 30, 60, **61**
  orthodromic form 60, 61–2, **65**, **67**,
    68, 123
  prognosis 66, 68
  therapy 68–9, 158–60
ACE inhibitors *see* angiotensin-
  converting enzyme (ACE) inhibitors
acebutolol 54, *141*
actinin genes 106
action potential *see* cardiac action
  potential
acute arrhythmias
  irregular 133–6
  narrow complex regular 121–8
  wide complex regular 128–33
adenosine
  diagnosis of DAD 16
  induction of AV block 123, 126, **127**
  mechanisms of action 16, 72, *138*,
    142, *144*
  RVOT 16, 72, **73**
adenosine-sensitive tachycardia *see*
  right ventricular outflow tract
  tachycardia
adenylate cyclase 72
after depolarisations 10, **14**, 15–16, 72,
  100–1, *138*
alcohol intake 116
alinidine *144*
ambulatory electrocardiography *see*
  Holter monitoring
amiodarone 82, 110, *139*, *141*, 142,
  144, 145
  adverse effects 147–8
  atrial fibrillation 52, 53, **54**, 55

atrial tachycardia 34
  cardiomyopathies 90, 92
  interactions 148
  ventricular tachycardia 85
anatomic re-entrant circuits 22–3, **24**
  atrial flutter 36, **39**
  atrial tachycardia 34–6
aneurysm, right ventricular 106
angiography 81–2, 108–9
angiotensin-converting enzyme (ACE)
  inhibitors 90
anisotropic propagation 21
anisotropic re-entry 25–6
antiarrhythmic drugs
  author's approach to 146–7
  interactions 148
  mechanisms of action 137–40
  proarrhythmic effects 142, 145–6,
    150
  Sicilian Gambit classification 142,
    143–4
  site-specific (Touboul) classification
    141–2
  Vaughan Williams classification
    140–1
  see also individual drugs
Antiarrhythmics versus Implantable
  Defibrillators (AVID) trial 161,
  163, **165**, 167
anticonvulsant agents *146*
antidepressants *146*
antihistamines *146*
antimicrobial agents *146*
antipsychotic agents *146*
arrhythmogenic right ventricular
  cardiomyopathy/dysplasia (ARVD)
  104–11
  anatomy 106
  background 104
  characteristics and mechanisms
    109–10

170